Marvin D. Feit, PhD
Stanley F. Battle, PhD
Editors

Health and Social Policy

Pre-publication
REVIEWS,
COMMENTARIES,
EVALUATIONS . . .

"**T**his book is a must for both practitioners and students in the field of health, welfare, and public health social work. For the practitioner, this book provides current information which examines several important issues of our day. For the practitioner and the student, the book provides several contributions that explore the interaction of health and welfare in depth. Further, there is diversity among the issues under examination as well as among the gender, cultures, and socioeconomic status of populations reviewed. . . . I highly recommend this important book."

Oliver J. Williams, MPH, PhD
Graduate School of Social Work
University of Minnesota

More pre-publication
REVIEWS, COMMENTARIES, EVALUATIONS . . .

"This book, *Health and Social Policy*, represents a major contribution for those scholars, health and social welfare planners, and human service advocates interested in the interplay between current social welfare and health policy issues. The editors and authors have done an excellent job of bridging the gap between areas of social welfare and health policy. The problems and issues have been presented with a great deal of clarity.

The book, with its excellent group of scholarly articles, is quite relevant and timely in that it addresses the major issues–such as AIDS, the homeless, and the uninsured–related to social welfare and health policy currently being debated in the United States. Furthermore, it offers an interdisciplinary overview of these all-important issues.

Finally, the book represents a fresh approach in looking comprehensively at a set of issues related to health and welfare that historically have been viewed as though they were separate entities."

Edward A. McKinney, MPH, PhD
Professor of Social Work
Cleveland State University,
Cleveland, OH

"This is an excellent volume which is very successful in dealing with the interface of social policy and health policy. The health planning section of the volume is particularly noteworthy. Chapters in this section range from assessments of Medicare's prospective payment system to an examination of need projection methodologies as an approach to implementing health planning policies for the 1990s.

The book's section on population issues is outstanding. It includes very useful essays on the potential family role of low income, adolescent, minority fathers and the need for providing formal and informal supports for such fathers. This section also includes an excellent study of the importance of family, the yin-yang philosophy of health care, and modesty concerns which must be taken into account when providing medical treatment for many Asian immigrant families.

The Haworth Press, Inc.

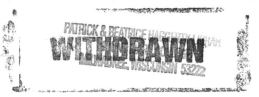

Health and Social Policy

HAWORTH Health and Social Policy
Marvin D. Feit, PhD
Senior Editor

New, Recent, and Forthcoming Titles:

Maltreatment and the School-Age Child: Developmental Outcomes and System Issues by Phyllis T. Howing, John S. Wodarski, P. David Kurtz, and James Martin Gaudin, Jr.

Health and Social Policy edited by Marvin D. Feit and Stanley F. Battle

Adolescent Substance Abuse: An Empirical-Based Group Preventive Health Paradigm by John S. Wodarski and Marvin D. Feit

Health
and Social Policy

Marvin D. Feit, PhD
Stanley F. Battle, PhD
Editors

The Haworth Press
New York • London • Norwood (Australia)

The Haworth Press, Inc., 10 Alice Street, Binghamton, NY 13904-1580

Library of Congress Cataloging-in-Publication Data

Feit, Marvin D.
    Health and social policy / Marvin D. Feit, Stanley F. Battle.
        p.   cm.
    Includes bibliographical references and index.
    ISBN 1-56024-343-0 (acid-free paper).
    1. Medical policy–United States. 2. Social medicine–United States. I. Battle, Stanley F. II. Title.
RA395.A3F45 1994
362.1'0973–dc20

93-6093
CIP

CONTENTS

ABOUT THE EDITORS

Marvin D. Feit, PhD, is Professor and Director of the School of Social Work at the University of Akron, Ohio. He has designed and taught courses in health and social policy and was Chair of a Health Substantive area. He is Co-Editor of *Evaluation of Employee Assistance Programs* (The Haworth Press, Inc.) and *Social Work Practice with the Elderly,* and the author of *Management and Administration of Drug and Alcohol Programs* as well as several book chapters and journal articles in the field of health and social work. Founding Co-Editor of the *Journal of Health & Social Policy,* he is a member of the National Association of Social Workers, the Council on Social Work Education, and the Association for the Advancement of Social Group Work.

Stanley F. Battle, PhD, is Associate Dean for Research & Development and Professor of Policy, Planning, and Research at the University of Connecticut School of Social Work, where he also has an appointment in the School of Medicine. Dr. Battle has designed and taught courses in Schools of Public Health, Social Work, and Medicine. He has edited, co-authored, and written six books and published over fifty academic articles. A member of the American Public Health Association, Dr. Battle is founding Co-Editor of the *Journal of Health & Social Policy* and serves as a contributing editor to *Social Work Research and Abstracts.*

Contributors

Jan Atwood, PhD, is affiliated with the College of Nursing and Arizona Cancer Center, University of Arizona.

Jayasree Basu, PhD, is Assistant Director and Chief of Methodology Development Research and Information Division, Maryland Health Resources Planning Commission, Department of Health and Mental Hygiene, 4201 Patterson Avenue, Baltimore, MD.

Stanley F. Battle, PhD, is Associate Professor of Policy and Planning, University of Connecticut, School of Social Work, 1798 Asylum Avenue, West Hartford, CT.

Chwee Lye Chng, PhD, is Associate Professor, Division of Kinesiology, Health Promotion and Recreation, University of North Texas, Denton, TX.

David C. Congdon, PhD, is affiliated with Norfolk State University, 2401 Corprew Avenue, School of Social Work, Norfolk, VA.

John Dobrowolsky, MSW, MBA, is Manager, Victoria Hospital, Family Medical Centre, 1244 Commissioners Road, London, Ontario, Canada.

Kathleen Ell, DSW, is Associate Professor, School of Social Work, University of Southern California and Director, The Rita and Maurice Hamovitch Social Work Research Center at the University of Southern California.

Marvin D. Feit, PhD, is Professor and Director of the School of Social Work, University of Akron, OH.

Wilbur Finch, DSW, is Associate Professor, School of Social Work, University of Southern California.

Frederick Fridinger, DrPH, is Associate Professor, Division of Kinesiology, Health Promotion and Recreation, University of North Texas, Denton, TX.

Deborah L. Fritz, PhD, is Executive Director of The Center for Prepaid Health Care Research in Rockville, MD, 1010 Grandin Avenue, #11, Rockville, MD.

John A. Garcia, PhD, is affiliated with the Mexican American Studies and Research Center, University of Arizona.

Marian Goldstein, ACSW, is Associate Director, Social Work Services, LIJ Division, Long Island Jewish Medical Center, New Hyde Park, NY.

Judith T. Gonzalez, PhD, is affiliated with the Mexican American Studies and Research Center, University of Arizona.

Stephen J. Gould, PhD, is Assistant Professor of Marketing at Rutgers, The State University of New Jersey.

Jan L. Hagen, PhD, ACSW, is Associate Professor, School of Social Welfare, Nelson A. Rockefeller College of Public Affairs and Policy, University at Albany, State University of New York, 135 Western Avenue, Albany, NY.

Michael J. Holosko, PhD, is Associate Professor, School of Social Work, University of Windsor, Windsor, Ontario.

Marybeth Hopkins, CSW, is Social Work Research Coordinator, Department of Social Work Services, Hillside Hospital, a division of Long Island Jewish Medical Center, New Hyde Park, NY.

Woodrow Jones is affiliated with the Department of Political Science, Texas A&M University, College Station, TX.

Neela P. Joshi, MD, is affiliated with the Departments of Pediatrics, Boston University School of Medicine and The Fallon Clinic, 630 Plantation Street, Worcester, MA.

Verna M. Keith is affiliated with the Department of Sociology, Texas A&M University, College Station, TX.

Patricia A. Keimig, MA, is Director of Health Systems Planning, Maryland Health Resources Planning Commission, Department of Health and Mental Hygiene, 4201 Patterson Avenue, Baltimore, MD.

Susan K. Kutzner, PhD, RN, is Adjunct Assistant Professor in the Dept. of OB/GYN at Baylor College of Medicine. She is also a Visiting Professor at Texas Woman's University, College of Nursing and currently in private practice.

David Larson, MD, MSPH, is Research Psychiatrist, National Institute of Mental Health, Rockville, MD.

Frank L. Meyskens, MD, is affiliated with the Department of Internal Medicine, Arizona Cancer Center, University of Arizona.

Robert Nishimoto, DSW, is Assistant Professor, School of Social Work, University of Southern California.

Patricia A. Nolan, MD, MPH, is currently Director of the Pima County Health Department, located in Tucson, AZ. She is also a member of the adjunct faculty of the University of Arizona College of Medicine, in the Department of Family and Community Medicine.

Elizabeth B. Quitkin is Social Work Manager, Department of Social Work Services, Long Island Jewish Division, Long Island Jewish Medical Center, New Hyde Park, NY.

Mitchell F. Rice, PhD, is Professor of Public Administration and Political Science at Louisiana State University, Baton Rouge.

Barry Rock, DSW, is Director, Department of Social Work Services, Long Island Jewish Medical Center, New Hyde Park, NY.

Fred Sattler, MD, is Associate Professor of Medicine, University of Southern California and Coordinator, Interdisciplinary AIDS Service at Los Angeles County-University of Southern California Medical Center.

Michael M. O. Seipel, PhD, is Assistant Professor in the School of Social Work, Brigham Young University, Provo, UT.

Peggy B. Smith, PhD, is Professor in the Dept. of OB/GYN at Baylor College of Medicine, One Baylor Plaza, Houston, TX. She is also Director, Teen Health Clinic, Jefferson Davis Hospital.

Preface

This text combines the separate fields of health and social welfare. The major interdisciplinary point of connection is policy, and the articles in this text illustrate the complex nature of this connection. It is our contention that one cannot separate health and social welfare issues in order to plan and work effectively in this field; although understanding each field separately may take many years of specialization. Further, it is difficult to appreciate the range of problems that emerge from each area.

Texts normally address health policy or social policy issues separately. The numerous problems related to each field, and their complexity, allow for texts to be written on each subject. Yet it is the interplay between both fields that often yields a whole new set and range of problems that health planners and/or social planners often overlook or rarely have an opportunity to handle effectively.

It is important to emphasize that when problems in health and social policy are combined a new and different set of problems and issues are highlighted. For example, screening for AIDS may make sense from the health perspective, while stigmatizing individuals from a social perspective. Drug testing may make sense for companies trying to demonstrate to an anxious public that they have a problem under control, however, as a screening mechanism, drug testing may or may not indicate the presence of a serious problem. In a third example, there may be every reason to believe that physicians are acting appropriately when they make heroic efforts to save the life of an elderly individual, yet from a social perspective questions arise regarding the allocation of resources and whether this the most appropriate way to spend needed health dollars.

These examples do not involve health or social policy issues alone; they combine in an intricate and dynamic manner in such a way that the public and professional debates become complex and appear unresolvable. Debates occur over a period of time in order that a favored position emerges. Positions are likely to change over time, while debates may arise periodically with differing outcomes.

This book provides a backdrop for the complexity of these issues. The authors highlight some of the problems that health and social planners might be expected to face as they develop programs and/or resolve some of the issues emerging from the interface of health and social welfare.

Some of the tension created by this interface is resolved by trying to achieve a sense of balance between health and social policy issues. In striving for this balance public attitude becomes a "wild" card. Public attitude often helps resolve issues by tipping the balance or acknowledging the range of problems that seem important at a particular time. For example, the push for increasing drug screens has come about because public attitude dictates the importance for companies to demonstrate they are doing something about the drug problem in this country. This means that the public may approve of a certain action because it wants a specific outcome, without really understanding some of the health issues and consequences. The action symbolizes or supports the public perception that officials are listening to them.

The fact that there are differential responses to different population groups and their problems is often a factor in helping to "tip" the balance toward a resolution of difficult issues. In some cases with minority or politically impotent groups the differential use of resources is most vividly seen with social factors playing a very important part in the allocation of health and medical resources. For example, in renal dialysis it is often clear that African Americans do not receive the same amount of resources as white Americans do, despite the need.

There are many other examples, but it is extremely important to note that social factors influence the way in which health and medical resources are allocated. Also, the complexity of the interaction between health and social policy issues creates new issues and problems that others have to address. Another dimension of public influence is that what is important today may not be tomorrow.

The public's attitude and response toward treating people with AIDS will continue to shift according to who is identified as the affected population. At first the public's perception was that AIDS was predominantly and almost exclusively a gay and minority problem. However, in the past couple of years the affected population has shifted to include heterosexual people. This shift is likely to bring about a different response by the public, and provide additional money for research and treatment.

By definition, issues generally pose problems for specific groups in society when the answers may be many or not easily attainable. For example, there is a battle cry for health care reform today. The demand for reform seems to increase as the number of problems with the current health care system continue to mount in number and severity. However, while solutions have been proposed none have been enacted on a national level because there is no agreement as to which one is favored by the public. For example, in the current health care debate the public remains confused over the total cost for reform solutions, the significant problems that may result from health care reform, or the need for health care reform itself. One is confused because it is not clear what is considered adequate medical care, how much money each proposed solution will actually cost, which services are to be offered, and so forth. The complexity of the problem is heightened by a combination of health policy concerns and social implications. Thus, an important issue such as health care reform is not simply a health and medical problem, but is underscored by the significant range of problems in the social and economic arena.

It is problematic that issues usually have no definitive solutions because there are no specific answers upon which to guide the planner or to give some direction to an anxious public. The resolution of health care reform will probably await the direction by the public as to what they'll settle for and what they think is most important. Helping to shape the public's perspective are numerous presentations in TV, radio, newspaper, printed magazines, and so forth. These presentations offer a particular viewpoint or agenda. What is most interesting in regard to health care reform is that the many problems and solutions are so numerous and confusing that all of this information seems to overwhelm the American public. Instead of mobilizing people around particular outcomes, the information appears to immobilize the public. Thus, this issue remains unresolved in part because there is no particular direction being taken at the present time.

For health care workers trying to plan and provide services, they must constantly deal with issues for which the answers are not readily or easily resolvable. This means they must work in a field with much uncertainty and at times not much direction. Workers may feel uneasy or uncomfortable about a proposed solution or direction because it may be unpopular or present problems not yet clearly understood. For example, if a politician selects a course of action that the public does not like, he or she may lose an election. Thus, it is very difficult for planners and other workers in the health and social welfare field to develop plans upon which they feel comfortable proposing to a waiting public. Much inaction is likely to occur because a consensus has not been reached.

A critical factor, illustrated in this book, is that effective outcomes require an understanding of policy issues and problems inherent in both the health and social welfare fields. This seems to present another area of concern and study because our educational process in each field is to treat these matters separately. However, this book illustrates the complex nature of the range of problems that exist in the combined field of health and social welfare. For example, Nolan illustrates the structural conflicts between the health and welfare systems that often hinder poor people from receiving prevention information and preventive care even though this is a medical and public health desired outcome. Also, while the health care strategies that affect Asian Americans are highlighted, the article raises questions about designing health care strategies as they impact upon various minority groups or ethnic groups. Likewise, when one examines changing family roles or adolescent fathers one is also illustrating how social problems can often identify the need for serving this population in the health field. Adolescent fathers may affect the medical outcome of the mother and the newborn, thus better health care outcomes may be obtained by including health initiatives with the social dimensions of family and family care.

In each of the articles selected one finds strain between social and public policy and health and medical intervention. As important, is that no easy answers are available. Thus, the focus in this text is to illustrate the problem, document the situation and highlight the issue. It is not easy to discern answers for a particular population Nevertheless, allocation of resources are made, programs are developed, and people continue to be provided services. One question raised in this text is whether health care workers are able to understand the complexity of the issues before them and be willing to engage other professionals in bringing about a more fair and just situation. In policy making there are no definitive answers. Outcomes are not always clear. There are competing vested interests, cost is often a factor not easily understood by the participants, and implementation of solutions often result in conflicts between competing organizations or between competing groups. It is with this knowledge that we encourage readers who are examining health and social welfare issues to read the articles in order to gain an appreciation of the complexity of their interface. Offered is not a prescription to follow, but to use the articles as a sample of the problems and issues one typically will be called upon to address. We believe that the authors will help the reader understand the complexity of the policy-making process and policy implementation in this field.

In summary this text is designed to illustrate the complex nature of the interface between the health and social welfare field. While often there are no definitive answers to many problems it is important for one to understand that services are continuing to be provided and money is continuing to be allocated in this ever-increasing area of service need. Our position is clear. This field is far too complex to leave it to the separate province of either social planners or health planners. It is important that the planning and the development of resources should consider the nature of the problems existing in both fields and as they interact with one another. The text may give some clue as to how to best design programs and illustrate some difficulties in planning methodologies for the programs. It is only when one understands the forces that act upon each other, thereby creating another new set of issues and problems to be addressed, that we will move toward a better system of care and a better system of providing services to a broader number of affected individuals in this country.

PUBLIC POLICY ISSUES

Despite significant differences in ideology, values, and social organization, most Western nations face common problems in developing appropriate policy to serve the poor on a national and local level. As populations at risk demand more medical care, there is a growing concern in the United States to provide a minimal level of service to all and to decrease obvious inequalities. In the United States we tend to use health care as the last line of defense for populations at great risk. Primary prevention for many is a luxury; as a result there is a tendency to link existing preventive services to defined groups. We seem to focus our attention on more economic ways of providing primary preventive services to groups at risk without too great an emphasis on follow up. This section will examine HIV antibody testing; medical indigency; inner city hospital care; determinants of health services utilization among the elderly; and options for providing health care for the uninsured.

Chapter 1

HIV Antibody Testing:
Who Benefits and Who Loses?

Chwee Lye Chng
Frederick Fridinger

SUMMARY. From a public health perspective, a significant milestone in the AIDS crisis has been the development of serologic tests to detect exposure to the HIV. AIDS is now reported in more than 124 countries and in every state of the Union. With the possibility that in excess of two million Americans have been infected, and in the absence of a cure or vaccine, the issue of testing cannot be ignored. Unfortunately, the testing debate has generated more heat than light. This chapter examines the proposed "benefit" to public health in testing target groups deemed "at risk," and also discusses socio-ethical implications of such testing. HIV antibody testing raises the need for a balance between voluntary and mandatory testing and forces society to reexamine commitment to protect public health while safeguarding individual civil rights.

INTRODUCTION

"Testing" for AIDS has considerable appeal today. AIDS is now reported in more than 124 countries and in every state of the Union. With the possibility that in excess of two million Americans have already been infected, and in the absence of a cure or vaccine, some politicians have called for mandatory HIV (Human Immuno-deficiency Virus) antibody testing (hereafter referred to as testing) to

This chapter was originally published in *Journal of Health & Social Policy*, Vol. 1(1) 1989.

help curb the spread of AIDS infection. Despite widespread opposition from the medical and civil rights communities to such universal testing, the White House has endorsed this measure. Unfortunately, the testing controversy has generated more heat than light.

Critics of mandatory testing have argued that such routine testing would not be financially, logistically, or ethically feasible. More important, testing would divert limited national resources away from education, treatment, and research; its immediate and potential costs would easily exceed its projected "benefits." Instead, health care professionals recommend voluntary and anonymous testing with appropriate counseling (Gostin & Curran, 1987). To them, anything more intrusive might alienate the very people a risk-reduction program is seeking to reach. These critics have interpreted the government's call for such widespread testing as another feeble attempt to give the illusion of decisive action–a "social placebo" designed to reassure a frightened people.

Unfortunately, rather than calming the public about the health crisis, the controversy generated over testing has raised unnecessary public concern and fear in people typically not deemed at risk. A poll conducted by *U.S. News and World Report* found that more than one in four adults in the United States worry that they might get AIDS (*U.S. News and World Report*, April 20, 1987).

This paper examines the controversy surrounding the policy of mandatory testing and discusses the need for a balance between voluntary and mandatory testing. It also examines the feasibility and benefit to public health in testing certain target groups deemed "at risk."

MANDATORY HIV ANTIBODY TESTING

The premise behind mandatory testing for HIV antibodies is twofold: (1) to encourage a change in sexual and other high-risk behaviors among the infected and at-risk individuals, and (2) to protect the uninfected from AIDS (McCusker et al., 1988). Some have suggested that knowledge of antibody status could lead inevitably to risk-reduction behavior. This assumption, however, has not been supported by empirical data. Since the spread of AIDS can only be reduced through the willingness of individuals not to engage in high-risk activities, the introduction of mandatory testing might be counter-productive (Fox, Odaka, & Polk, 1986). Testing would inevitably drive the people most in need away from the services they might otherwise seek: counseling and education about AIDS. In effect, mandatory testing would create an unnecessary and unhealthy adversarial relationship between the government and groups at risk.

In the absence of a vaccine or effective treatment for AIDS–and the lack of evidence that knowledge of serologic status would necessarily lead to positive behavioral changes–the only justification for mandatory testing is the protection of the uninfected. Does mandatory testing protect the general population? This question will be examined in the context of testing for exposure to the HIV in premarital couples, inmates of prisons, and insurance and job applicants.

Premarital Testing

Premarital testing has been proposed to help protect the uninfected spouse and future offsprings. Although only Texas, Louisiana and Illinois have passed such laws, similar legislation has been introduced in more than 30 other states. From a public health perspective premarital testing has limited value: it will do little to protect people from infection since marriage is not necessary for sexual intercourse or impregnation. Many people who marry will have sexual intercourse before marriage, so they could spread the HIV before testing. Also, it would be ineffective in stopping the spread of AIDS from mother to unborn children, because most infected babies have been born to unmarried mothers (Donovan, 1987). More important, a premarital screening requirement does not guarantee a change in the future sexual or reproductive behavior of a married couple. Ironically, the two largest groups of infected individuals, homosexual-bisexual males and intravenous drug users, are not the most likely applicants for a marriage license. Evidently, universal premarital testing will not have a significant impact on the spread of the infection.

The cost of managing such a large-scale program is prohibitive and incommensurate with the potential benefits. Nationwide mandatory premarital testing would detect fewer than one-tenth of one percent of infected people, at a cost of more than $100 million per year (Donovan, 1987). Of the more than 3.5 million people expected to get married in a typical year, mandatory premarital testing would detect only about 1,200 infected people who have not already transmitted the HIV to their partners (U.S. Dept. of Commerce, 1986). Besides the cost for the ELISA and confirmatory tests, there are the expenses associated with personnel for counseling and laboratory work, laboratory and office space, and printed materials.

When used with low-risk groups such as premarital couples, the potential for false-positives and false-negatives would be unacceptably high. In an age where persons with AIDS or the HIV antibodies, and even people "perceived" to be at risk for AIDS, have been victims of discrimination, the marginal public health benefit of premarital screening does not justify its high social cost. High-risk individuals or those interested in knowing their antibody status can voluntarily and anonymously be tested.

Testing in Prison

The spread of AIDS in prisons has caused concern. The problem is likely to increase in light of the growing number of inmates who have been intravenous drug users prior to incarceration, and the level of sexual activity that takes place in prison (Glass et al., 1988). More than half of all prison deaths in the New York state correctional system are AIDS-related (Berkmoes, 1986). To date, there are over 1,000 cases of AIDS in state prisons, with an estimated 21,000 to 42,000 inmates infected with the HIV (Vaid, 1985). In June 1987, the nation's federal prison system initiated mandatory testing of incoming and outgoing inmates. Several states now routinely segregate inmates with AIDS, ARC, or HIV antibodies (Glass et al., 1988).

Most prison systems test inmates if they show symptoms. Three states (Colorado, Nevada, and South Dakota) have already instituted mandatory testing of all inmates (Vaid, 1985). Given that prisons are already overcrowded, the cost of housing seropositive inmates in separate quarters would be prohibitive. It is unclear whether mandatory testing would result in better health protection for the prison population. Mandatory, universal testing may result in problems ranging from unequal facilities and treatment to potential violence and discrimination. Isolation of seropositive inmates is only justifiable if the inmate represents a real danger to others. Testing positive on the ELISA is not the same as having AIDS or spreading the infection. Inmates with AIDS, ARC, or HIV antibodies are often segregated from others, ostensibly to protect them from violence, rather than to protect the prison population from infection. The legality and morality of such segregations are questionable. From a public health perspective, segregating all infected inmates together will provide opportunities for unprotected sexual intercourse and IV drug use which may eventually precipitate a health crisis in the prison system. Testing and segregation can give a false sense of security. The test does not identify infected individuals who have not seroconverted. These false-negatives continue to pose a real public health risk to the prison population.

Mandatory testing is intrusive, unnecessary, expensive, and ineffective. More important, it does not address the means of AIDS transmission in prison—consensual or forcible homosexual intercourse and intravenous drug use among inmates. Because of the criminal and moral prohibitions of these two activities, many prison systems are still reluctant to circulate condoms among inmates or provide explicit AIDS education (ACLU, 1986). Protection of inmates against rape and a reduction of IV drug use would certainly produce more public health benefits than mass testing.

Mandatory testing has implications both inside and outside the prison system. It unnecessarily jeopardizes the inmate's privacy by the gathering of highly personal and potentially incriminating information, which if disclosed would not only stigmatize the inmate, but could seriously damage prospects of rehabilitation upon release. For after all, in the minds of many people AIDS is still closely associated with such socially disapproved phenomena as homosexuality and drug use. Even former Attorney General Meese has stated publicly that HIV infection should be a factor in parole eligibility for incarcerated persons. In effect, he is saying that people exposed to HIV truly belong in prison.

In light of the socio-cultural context in which mandatory testing of all inmates has been proposed, not only will it not curb the spread of infection, it can potentially cause more social problems on both sides of the prison wall. Mandatory testing neither protects the prison population nor promotes positive behavioral change. On the other hand, voluntary anonymous testing with appropriate counselling and explicit AIDS education of all inmates and prison staff would be more beneficial.

Testing of Insurance Applicants

The controversy surrounding testing insurance applicants stems from the high health care costs of persons with AIDS and ARC (ranging from $28,000 to $147,000), and its potential impact on the course of medical diagnosis and treatment in the country. It is further compounded by the groups at high risk who are also politically unpopular and economically vulnerable: homosexual and bisexual males, and intravenous drug users.

Primarily AIDS has struck males between the ages of 20 and 50–a large cohort found in company-sponsored health insurance group policies that until recently had experienced the lowest rates of utilization. In this regard, AIDS has struck at the very heart of underwriting. Because of the enormous costs involved, some carriers are screening applicants for the HIV antibodies and denying them coverage; others have "dumped" AIDS patients or rejected their claims, stating they were "pre-existing conditions," a position seldom taken with other life-threatening conditions (Levine & Joyce, 1985). Still others have attempted to exclude AIDS from coverage on new policies.

From a public health perspective, this position of the insurance industry is untenable since, in effect, it actively discourages even voluntary testing among members of high-risk groups. Individuals concerned about their health in light of the potential economic ramifications may not want to risk their insurability in order to know their serologic status. Furthermore, while testing may have some actuarial value if used prudently, it is a very imprecise and unreliable means of predicting who will eventually contract AIDS.

Maine and the District of Columbia recognized these adverse public health implications of testing and have, for the time being, prohibited insurers from requiring anyone to take the test or inquiring if they have had such a test. They also restrict insurers from basing rates or other aspects of coverage by whether the applicant has taken such a test (Faden & Kass, 1988). Before testing of insurance applicants is permitted, steps must be taken to eliminate the negative consequences of testing. Minimally, confidentiality of insurance records, including test results, must be strengthened and legal protection against discrimination must also be in effect. Past presidents (Reagan and Bush) have gone on record that they would oppose any legislation that protects against discrimination of persons with AIDS, ARC, or HIV antibodies and that guarantees confidentiality of testing results. This stated opposition to federal confidentiality protections ironically conflicts with the Administration's call for mandatory testing.

Proponents for mandatory testing of insurance applicants argue that early identification and exclusion of infected applicants is needed to protect an insurer's solvency. Despite such publicized fears, there is no documented evidence that insurance carriers are at greater risk of insolvency as a direct result of AIDS-related claims. There is, however, a substantial risk to those tested which may result in a denial of employment, housing, loans, and credits.

Insurance companies, therefore, must have a justifiable medical basis for requiring a test. Simply being a homosexual male should not be regarded as a negative underwriting factor or a proxy variable for positive HIV results, but engaging in high-risk sexual practices should. Behavior, not status, places a person at risk. Where needed, anonymous testing is preferred to other forms of testing, and written informed consent should always be sought. To further protect applicants, it is imperative that a confirmatory test should follow initial ELISA tests before any actuarial decision is made.

CONCLUSION

In the absence of a cure or vaccine, it would be futile to identify those exposed to the HIV; it would be better to educate everyone about the risks, irrespective of their age, sex, race, or sexual preference. The most effective means of limiting the spread of AIDS is not through mandatory testing but by encouraging high-risk individuals to seek testing on their own, to protect them from subsequent discrimination, and to help them change their high-risk behaviors (Becker & Joseph, 1988). As education continues, the stigma of AIDS should lessen considerably. In time, more people may be willing not only to be tested for exposure to the HIV, but also to make behavioral changes to limit the spread of AIDS.

REFERENCES

American Civil Liberties Union. (1986). National Prison Project status report on prison. Feb. 20.

Becker, M., & Joseph, J. (1988). AIDS and behavioral change to reduce risk: A review. *American Journal of Public Health*, 78(4), 394-410.

Berkmoes, R. (1986). AIDS deaths fuel concern of spread in jails. *American Medical News*, 29,7.

Donovan, P. (1987). AIDS and family planning clinics: Confronting the crisis. *Family Planning Perspective*, 19(3), 111-138.

Faden, R., & Kass, N. (1988). Health insurance and AIDS: The status of state regulatory activity. *American Journal of Public Health*, 78(4), 437-438.

Fox, R., Odaka, N., & Polk, B. (1986). *Effect of learning HTLV-III/LAV antibody status on subsequent sexual activity*. Proceedings of the 2nd International AIDS Conference, Paris.

Glass, G., Hausler, W., Loeffelholz, P., & Yesalis III, C. (1988). Seroprevalence of HIV Antibody among individuals entering the Iowa prison system. *American Journal of Public Health*, 78(4), 447-449.

Gostin, L., & Curran, W. (1987). AIDS screening, confidentiality, and the duty to warn. *American Journal of Public Health*, 77(3), 361-365.

Levine, C., & Joyce, B. (Eds.) (1985). AIDS: The emerging ethical dilemma. *Hastings Center Report Special Supplement*, 15(4), Hastings-on-Hudson, NY: Hastings Center.

McCusker, J., Stoddard, A., Mayer, K., Zapka, J., Morrison, C., Saltzman, S. (1988). Effects of HIV antibody test knowledge on subsequent sexual behaviors in a cohort of homosexual active men. *American Journal of Public Health*, 78(4), 462-467.

U.S. Department of Commerce. (1986). *Bureau of the Census: Statistical abstract of the United States* (106th ed.).

U.S. News and World Report. April 20, 1987. 56-59.

Vaid, U. (1985). National Prison Project gathers the facts on AIDS in prison. *ACLU National Prison Project, Winter*, 1-6.

Chapter 2

Medical Indigency
and Inner City Hospital Care:
Patient Dumping, Emergency Care,
and Public Policy

Mitchell F. Rice

SUMMARY. This chapter discusses the growing lack of private for-profit hospital care for the medically indigent. The issues of patient dumping and emergency care are examined from both judicial and public policy perspectives. The chapter concludes by noting that dumping may be viewed as a most serious form of neglect and more comprehensive laws and court decisions are needed to require all hospitals, regardless of ownership, to treat all patients who arrive at their doors if the hospitals have the appropriate medical staff and facilities.

INTRODUCTION

Changes in financing of the American health care system during the last few years have resulted in major gaps in the "safety net" which protects the poor/indigent from the ravages of disease and illness. These changes have favored a shift toward market competitiveness as a means of controlling rising health care costs. As this

The author wishes to acknowledge research assistance provided by graduate student Carl Primeaux.

This chapter was originally published in *Journal of Health & Social Policy*, Vol. 1(2) 1989.

approach has become more characteristic of the American health care system, the problems of the medically indigent have become more pronounced. The severity of medical indigency has led some 30 states to establish task forces to study the problem. Nowhere is the problem more acute than in the growing lack of private for-profit hospital care for the medically indigent. About two-thirds of the hospitals in the country are private institutions.

Public and/or charity hospital use has been on an increase in recent years. This increase can be attributed to several factors: (1) changes in Medicaid eligibility requirements; (2) changes in Medicare reimbursement schedules; (3) a general increase in the number of uninsured individuals; and (4) the alarming increase in the transfer of uninsured and underinsured patients from private for-profit hospitals to public/charity hospitals, a phenomenon known as "dumping." Other terminologies used to describe this phenomenon are "case shifting" and "economically motivated transfers" (Duncan and Vogel, 1988).

Hospital dumping has generated considerable attention in both the health and political arenas. The attention has magnified because of the increasing number of transfer patients requiring emergency care upon arrival at a public hospital. In some cases private for-profit hospitals have delayed treatment or flatly refused to treat uninsured or underinsured individuals. As a result, the death or permanent disability of patients has occurred ("Hospitals in Cost Squeeze," 1985; Klaidman, 1986; Wren, 1985; Friedman, 1982; Editorial, 1982). Yet, for years the transfer of patients from one hospital to another had been considered appropriate (and still is) when patients need special care and/or services that are unavailable at the referring hospital.

On February 5, 1985 and February 6, 1985, *CBS Evening News* and *ABC Evening News*, respectively, reported the following incident. A 34-year-old (uninsured black man) with a wound from a knife which penetrated his skull, was denied emergency neurosurgery at a private hospital. Though the hospital began treatment in the emergency room, and had complete neurosurgical facilities, the patient was refused further care. Following transfer to another facility (two other hospitals refused to accept him) the patient died.

In other cases private for-profit hospitals have provided only a modicum of care to stabilize the patient for transfer to a public hospital. Upon arrival the patient's health had deteriorated to such a point that death or permanent disability occured. In Chicago, for example, nearly 25 percent of the transfers to Cook County Hospital were in unstable condition and their death rate was two and one-half times higher than that of other patients (Trafford et al., 1986). Further, in areas where indigency or public aid is not accepted as a reason for transfer, a transferring hospital may often misrepresent the reason for transfer. A hospital may claim the transfer is purely for a medical reason.

Why do private for-profit hospitals transfer (dump) uninsured and underinsured patients to public hospitals? Do private for-profit hospitals have legal and moral obligations to provide emergency care to all who seek their services? This chapter addresses these questions. These questions are especially noteworthy since the profit margin of the private hospital sector (at least in 1984) in the United States was at its highest in 20 years (Ansell and Schiff, 1987).[1] The chapter also discusses governmental policy responses to the dumping issue.

THE DUMPING PHENOMENON

Ansell and Schiff (1987:1500) define patient dumping "as the denial of or limitation in the provision of medical services to a patient for economic reasons and the referral of that patient elsewhere." Dumped patients can be divided into two categories: inpatient and outpatient.

> Inpatient dumping involves ambulatory hospital-to-hospital transfer of patients too sick to be discharged but stable enough to transfer. Outpatient dumping involves those patients who require hospitalization but who may safely be discharged (*Americans at Risk*, 1985:30-36, testimony by Dr. G. Schiff).

Outpatient dumping is difficult to quantify and study because there is little or no follow up of such patients. It is difficult to ascertain if an individual has been refused treatment as an outpatient at an emergency care facility.

While dumping can occur in any part of a hospital, it most commonly occurs in the emergency room. This is not surprising since emergency room use has risen rapidly in recent years. By 1984 some 160 million visits were expected to the emergency room. An increase of 151 million visits or 1800 percent since 1954 (Wing and Campbell, 1985). While up to 30 percent of a hospital's admissions may come from the emergency room (Wing and Campbell, 1985), by dumping unwanted emergency room patients a hospital may exercise judgment regarding who it will or will not treat. Dumping can result from both hospital policies and practices. Examples of hospital policies and practices may include requiring advance payment, refusing patients who don't have a physician on the hospital's staff, or refusing to accept Medicaid patients. For minorities, especially blacks, dumping has serious implications in health care. For large numbers of blacks, the hospital emergency room is the provider of last resort (Sager, 1983). Rice (1985/86:66) notes that:

> More often than not the . . . hospital's emergency department serves as the entry point into the health-care system for inner-city blacks and the poor. The emergency department acts as the primary care center, preventive care center, trauma center and intensive care center all at once for the indigent patient such as the feverish baby, the shooting victim, the high-risk pregnant mother, the premature neonate, the unwedded teenage mother and so on.

A recent study of 1,066 patients from 26 urban public hospitals in 12 states and the District of Columbia indicates that dumping has become a widespread phenomenon (McCormick, 1986). The study points out that at least 15 percent of emergency transfer patients to public hospitals qualify as dumping. Some hospital analysts suggest that this figure may be considerably higher. For example, in Washington, D.C. transfers from private hospitals to D.C. General Hospital increased from 169 to about 1000 annually between the years 1981 and 1984 (Greensberg, 1984). The number of transfers to Cook County Hospital in Chicago increased by more than five times between 1980 and 1983; from 1295 to 6769 (Schiff et al., 1986; Dowell, 1984).

In Texas dumping has been recently documented at more than 40 hospitals (Smith, 1986). While hospital dumping has been more pronounced in urban areas, it has been reportedly occurring in smaller cities and rural areas ("Hospitals in Cost Squeeze," 1985). Further, the rights of indigent patients are ignored when a private hospital makes a decision to transfer. At Cook County hospital only 6 percent of transferred patients provided written consent for transfer (Schiff et al., 1986).

In some states such as Texas, Florida, Tennessee, and Kentucky profit-oriented hospital chains have proliferated and acquired a large share of the market, and dumping has become an extremely serious problem (Relman, 1986). In Texas private hospitals amount to about one-third of the total hospitals in the state. Even a Medicaid recipient is not immune from dumping. A study of 467 patient transfers to Cook County Hospital found that 46 percent were recipients of public aid (Schiff et al., 1986). Another 46 percent had no insurance. Further, the study suggests that insurance status may be closely associated with race. Schiff et al. (1986) found that 89 percent of the transfers involve minorities (blacks and Hispanics). The study also estimated the cost of care provided by Cook County Hospital to the transferred patients at 3.35 million dollars of which nearly 3 million was nonreimbursable; minimum costs that the private transferring hospitals would not have received had they provided care. Extrapolated for all of 1983, the total cost shifted to Cook County Hospital through transfers was 24 million dollars.

Himmelstein, Woolhandler, and Harnly (1984), in a study of 458 patients transferred to the emergency department of Highland General Hospital in Oakland, California, found that about 63 percent had no insurance, 21 percent had Medicaid, and only 3 percent had private insurance. The study also found that a disproportionate number of transferred patients were minorities. Schiff et al. (1986) found that of 1021 patient transfers to the Dallas Parkland Memorial Hospital about 77 percent had no third-party insurance. Parkland Memorial spends some 10 million dollars annually on transferred indigent patients (Frank, 1985). Ansell and Schiff (1987:1500) estimated that "250,000 patients nationwide in need of emergency care annually are transferred for economic reasons . . . representing a cost of 1.04 billion dollars to public hospitals."

Because hospitals are finding it increasingly difficult to shift the costs from one segment of their patient population to another, Ewe Reinhardt (1985:2) notes that "the uninsured poor themselves [have] become the hot potatoes one hospital seeks to dump into the lap of another." Until recently hospitals had little difficulty in shifting unreimbursed costs to three other sources: (1) private health insurance carriers and patients; (2) charitable foundations and private donations; and (3) private pay patients. With the decline in philanthropic donations, hospitals can only shift costs to privately insured patients. These charitable donations have in recent years covered no more than 4 percent of total health care costs (Milligan, 1986). In 1981 hospital cost shifting to private insured pay patients amounted to nearly 5 billion dollars (Wehr, 1982). These costs are reflected in higher rates for employers who sponsor health insurance plans. A large number of individuals are insured at their workplaces. From 1977 to 1982 yearly payments by employers for health insurance benefits more than doubled from 33 billion to 78 billion dollars (Berg, 1983). Recent cost-containment strategies are reducing the hospital's ability to shift costs to the privately insured. With nowhere to shift the costs of unreimbursed care, hospitals dump uninsured individuals rather than absorb the costs themselves.

Some studies support the view that a primary reason for transfer is the inability of patients to pay. For example, research by Harvard Medical School doctors of 103 patients transferred from private hospitals to Highland General Hospital in Oakland, California showed that transfers jeopardized the patients in one-third of the cases but also that transfers were for economic reasons rather than patient care and "the transfers were a form of medical abuse" ("Hospitals in Cost Squeeze," 1985:33).

EXPLANATIONS FOR HOSPITAL DUMPING

One explanation for the increase in dumping is that fewer patients have private hospital insurance. It is estimated that some 37 million people (15 percent of the total population) do not have medical insurance, Medicaid, or Medicare (Tolchin, 1988). About one-third are children under 18 years of age (Inglehart, 1985) and nearly 3 million are between the ages of 55 and 64 (*Americans at*

Risk, 1985:1). Another 50 million individuals are underinsured (Reinhardt, 1985).

The large numbers of uninsured and underinsured have caused hospitals, mostly public and voluntary not-for-profit hospitals, to provide in 1985 9.5 billion dollars in free care (Brider, 1987). While dumping occurs in both urban and rural areas, it is most pronounced in large metropolitan areas, since this is where large numbers of uninsured patients are found.[2] In Chicago, for example, it is estimated that some 600,000 individuals (one of every 5 individuals) have no health insurance. In Illinois nearly 20 percent of the black and 25 percent of the Hispanic adult populations are uninsured (Marsh, 1988). Further, some 25 percent of the black population nationwide between the ages of 18-64 are uninsured (Bovbjerg and Kopit, 1986). Blacks represent about 17.3 percent or some 4 million of the total uninsured (Sulvetta and Swartz, 1986). Moreover, some 25 percent of all black children are uninsured and black children comprise some 20 percent or 2.2 million of all uninsured children under 18 years of age (Sulvetta and Swartz, 1986).

Patient dumping has been exacerbated by changes in Medicaid eligibility requirements. President Reagan's budget pressures have significantly reduced the number of individuals covered by Medicaid. In 1984 Medicaid covered only some 38 percent of the poor, compared with some 65 percent in 1976 (Brider, 1987).[3] With the enactment of the Omnibus Budget Reconciliation of 1981 (Public Law 97-35), Medicaid was reduced by some 12.8 billion dollars. In 1982 with the enactment of the Tax Equity and Fiscal Responsibilities Act (Public Law 97-248), Medicaid was reduced by another 2.2 billion dollars through fiscal year 1985.

Private for-profit hospitals find it financially unattractive to provide care to the underinsured or to those unable to pay. As a result, private for-profit hospitals attempt to limit the number of uninsured patients they serve. Recent literature is supportive of this point. Rowland and Davis' (1982) analysis of the Office of Civil Rights (United States Department of Health and Human Services) survey data on inpatient admissions practices show that for-profit hospitals provided care to only 6 percent of uninsured patients in 1981. This compares to nearly 17 percent at state and local government hospitals. Their analysis also shows that of all the for-profit hospitals included in the survey data, about 60 percent had less than 5 percent uninsured admissions.

A second explanation has to do with the recent change in the way Medicare reimburses hospitals for care provided to elderly and disabled individuals.[4] Instead of reimbursing hospitals for the actual costs of treating Medicare patients, the federal government now pays a set fee according to 467 "diagnostic related groups" or DRGs (Social Security Act of 1983, Public Law 98-21). In 1988 one national rate applied to all hospitals.

This new system, also referred to as a prospective payment system, has created a reverse effect on how hospitals treat and care for their patients (Pfeiffer and Christian, 1987). If a hospital spends less on a patient than the fixed reimbursed amount, it makes a profit. If the hospital spends more, it must absorb the loss. The incentive for hospitals is to treat the elderly or disabled patient as economically and quickly as possible–or not at all (Baldwin, 1985).

DRG abuses have been documented by several studies. A General Accounting Office study (1985) concludes that patients are being discharged from the hospital in a poorer state of health. Other studies report that the DRG System has led to increased transfers of Medicare patients to nursing homes and other extended care facilities with a greater level of debility at the time of transfer. Morrisey et al. (1988a), in an examination of patient discharge data from a national sample of 467 hospitals for the years 1980, 1983, 1984 and 1985, report that the proportion of Medicare patients transferred to post-hospital settings nearly doubled after implementation of the DRG System. Morrisey et al. (1988b) in a similar study of 501 hospitals, noted that the prospective system increased the rate of discharges to subacute facilities.

Evidence now suggests that some hospitals will clearly be disadvantaged by the DRG system. These hospitals will tend to be in rural areas (Mueller and Comer, 1987) and have greater indigent and free care burdens (Valda, 1983; Aaron, 1984). Thus, the prospect exists that these hospitals may no longer be financially willing to provide care to those unable to pay or who are covered under the DRG system (Mueller and Comer, 1987). Thus it seems that increased dumping is directly related to the financial problems facing Medicaid/Medicare. Ironically, these two programs were enacted some twenty years ago to reduce the dumping of elderly and poor patients into charity wards and public hospitals.

A third explanation for an increase in dumping can be associated with the growing movement toward competitive health care, a reliance on market forces to determine the cost of care. While little empirical research has documented the effects competition has on costs and services of health care providers, it is quite clear that competition means hospitals are less likely to offer charity care. In the words of an administrator of a public hospital:

> To be medically indigent in a competitive system is tantamount to being an outcast. [and] Never in human history has economic competition resulted in the just distribution of scarce and life sustaining resources. (Millenson, 1987)

Further, the competition strategy assumes that individuals can make informed decisions about hospital services. Yet, the medically indigent are the least likely to have the technical knowledge and varied experiences in medical care to make a useful judgment about hospital care. This is especially so because of the limited health and hospital care providers available to the medically indigent. Moreover, emergency care for trauma or sudden illness for the medically indigent must be sought from the hospital willing or obligated to provide care, ruling out any possibility of a search.

HOSPITAL EMERGENCY CARE
AND THE MEDICALLY INDIGENT

In 1973 a court observed in *Mercy Medical Center v. Winnebago Co.* that:

> It would shock the public conscience if a person in need of emergency aid would be turned down at the door of a hospital having emergency service because that person could not at that moment assure payment for the service.

However, the traditional legal rule has been that hospitals are not required by "common law duty" to admit every person seeking admission.[5] This rule can be traced to a longstanding principle of tort law which holds that a person is not legally obligated to help another person in distress (Wing and Campbell, 1985). Under common law a hospital cannot be held liable for *nonfeasance*–for failure to render aid–to one in peril since it had no duty to act.[6] The Alabama Supreme Court in the 1934 case of *Birmingham Baptist Hospital v. Crews*, in a seminal ruling, held that a private hospital owes no duty to accept an emergency patient not desired by it and it does not have to provide a reason for refusal.[7]

In *Crews* a two-year-old girl with diphtheria was provided initial treatment, but was sent home without further treatment; she later died. Wing and Campbell (1985:130) equate the *Crews* ruling to a "drowning man" hypothetical:

> Assume a man is drowning in a lake with no hope of rescue. Must a passer-by who can easily throw a rope and save the man's life do so? The common-law answer is theoretically 'no.'

Using a similar analogy Fine (1983) says:

> Like a competent swimmer who may let a child drown, . . . hospitals are under no legal duty to rescue . . . .

The general rule (common law) in *Crews* has been maintained by courts in *Hill v. Ohio County* (1971), *LeJeune Road Hospital, Inc. v. Watson* (1965), and in *Harper v. Baptist Medical Center-Princeton* (1976). In *Hill*, a Kentucky court held that a public hospital had no duty to admit a pregnant woman who was about to give birth. In *Watson* a Florida District Court of Appeals ruled that a private hospital may reject any patient that it does not desire. In *Harper*, the Alabama Supreme Court reaffirmed its ruling in *Crews* by holding that the hospital was under no duty to admit the patient even after treating and stabilizing the patient in the emergency room.

However, the general rule established in *Crews* has been modified in several other court decisions. The courts have applied the concepts of "gratuitous undertaking" and "implied admission" to establish when a hospital is obligated to provide emergency care. The gratuitous undertaking theory imposes an obligation on the hospital once it begins to administer care. By beginning to render aid to an injured party, a hospital commits itself to provide emergency services to any member of the public in need of such services (*Williams v. Hospital Authority of Hall Co.*, 1969). Once responsibility for the party's well-being is assumed a hospital cannot discontinue service if it increases the risk of harm to the party (Comment, 1974). Using the drowning man hypothetical in the gratuitous theory, Wing and Campbell (1985:130) make the following observation as applicable to *Crews*:

> Assume that the passer-by undertakes to save the drowning man and throws a rope. Will the law obligate him to complete the effort, or may he arbitrarily abandon the rescue? . . . The reasoning [may be applied here] that [an] aborted rescue has not changed the drowning man's lot–he is still a drowning man, no better, no worse–so the passer-by has not *increased* the risk of harm.

A few decades later Prosser (cited in Wing and Campbell, 1985:131) using the same hypothetical noted a change in reasoning and thus a change in liability:

> It seems very unlikely that any court will ever hold that one who has began to pull a drowning man out of the river after he has caught hold of the rope, without good reason, to abandon the attempt, walk away, and let him drown, merely because he was already in extremis before the effort had begun.

The case of *O'Neill v. Montefiore Hospital* (1960) reflects this newer legal view of the gratuitous undertaking theory. In *O'Neill* the plaintiff entered the hospital room complaining of severe arm pains and believed he was having a heart attack. Montefiore Hospital did not accept patients with his kind of insurance policy. The attending nurse, however, did call a physician who worked with that kind of insurance. The plaintiff was instructed to go home until morning. Upon arriving home the plaintiff died of a heart attack. While there was no pre-existing hospital/patient relationship, the court found the phone call made by the nurse could constitute a gratuitous undertaking.

The implied admission theory suggests that once a hospital begins treatment and care it has implicitly admitted the party and effectuated a hospital-patient contract (Comment, 1974). Each of these theories requires the performance of a specific act by a hospital which can be construed as an exercise of control over the patient. Court decisions in *New Biloxi Hospital, Inc. v. Frazier* (1962), *Methodist Hospital v. Ball,* (1961), *Fjerstad v. Knutson* (1978), and in *Hunt v. Palm Springs General Hospital* (1977) have advanced these theories. In *Frazier* (p. 197) the Mississippi Supreme Court outlined the hospital's duty to the patient:

> In an emergency, the victim should be permitted to leave the hospital only after he has been seen, examined and offered reasonable first aid. In undertaking to do so, a hospital must exercise due care. A hospital emergency treatment is obligated to do that which is immediately and reasonably necessary for the preservation of the life, limb or health of the patient. It should not discharge a patient in critical condition without furnishing or procuring suitable medical attention.

In *Fjerstad* (pp. 11-12) the Supreme Court of South Dakota provided the following interpretation of the undertaking theory.

> Although it has been held that a hospital, even one operating an emergency room, has no duty to accept a patient for treatment . . . once [a hospital] undertakes to render medical aid, the hospital is required to do so non-negligently. . . . The duty arose in this case, since the hospital undertook, through its nurses and intern, to render treatment to decedent. Decedent has a right to expect that the treatment rendered by a hospital which maintains and staffs an emergency room would be commensurate with that available in the same or similar communities or in hospitals generally.

While decisions in the more recent cases may be viewed as favoring the medically indigent, the decisions in the earlier cases leave the impact of case law on hospital behavior somewhat unclear. The decisions have not clearly established how and when patients status begins nor have they determined the criteria for hospital admission. On the one hand, the slightest undertaking on the part of the hospital can lead to a hospital/patient relationship. On the other hand, a hospital can flatly refuse to treat an individual and escape liability.

An alternate theory, used by several courts, holds a hospital liable for failure to render emergency care where an "unmistakable" emergency exists and the hospital has a well-established custom of rendering emergency services (*Wilmington General Hospital v. Manlove*, 1961). Stated another way, this view, also known as the reliance theory (Dowell, 1984), holds that a hospital which maintains an emergency room is inviting for treatment patients who have a need for emergency care. The Delaware Supreme Court held in *Manlove* that the hospital may be liable even though treatment was not undertaken. Using this reasoning, the court avoided the problem of finding an affirmative act to trigger liability under the gratuitous undertaking and implied admission theories. Yet, the *Manlove* decision does not clearly point out hospital liability and duty to treat. In *Manlove* the court did not define when an "unmistaken emergency" exists, when a hospital has a "well-established custom of providing emergency care" and when prospective patient has a "reliance" on the hospital's custom of providing emergency care.

Defining Medical Emergency
and Emergency Care

Until recently it was considered the social responsibility of a hospital to provide emergency care to those in need regardless of the ability to pay. In other words, to be treated in an emergency room for an emergency condition has been viewed as a secure non-statutory right; that is a right based on "the right to medical care" (Annas, 1986). Further, the public also considers the "emergency room as a neighborhood center, and expects it to provide around-the-clock primary care and emergency care with equal skill and speed" (Wing and Campbell, 1985:120). The general public definition of a medical emergency is "any illness or injury requiring immediate attention" (Dowell, 1984).

Similarly, national medical and physicians organizations also provide a broad definition of a medical emergency.

The American College of Surgeons has stated that "the function of an emergency department is to give adequate evaluation and initial treatment or advice to all persons who consider themselves acutely ill or injured and present themselves at the emergency room" (cited in Dowell, 1984). The American College of Emergency Physicians has defined a medical emergency as:

1. any condition resulting in admission of the patient to a hospital or nursing home within 24 hours;
2. evaluation or repair of acute (less than 72 hours) trauma;
3. relief of acute or severe pain;
4. investigation or relief of acute infection;
5. protection of public health;
6. obstetrical crises and/or labor;
7. hemorrhage or treatment of hemorrhage;
8. shock or impending shock; . . .
13. any sudden and/or serious symptom(s) which might indicate a condition which constitutes a threat to the patient's physical or psychological well-being requiring immediate medical attention to prevent possible deterioration, disability, or death. (cited in Dowell, 1984:484)

In some cases the courts have based their decisions on the emergency care policy provisions of national hospital and medical associations. In *Guerrero v. Copper Queen Hospital* (1975), the Arizona Court of Appeals relied on the emergency care provision of the Joint Commission on the Accreditation of Hospitals (1984) which states:

Any individual who comes to the hospital for emergency medical evaluation or initial treatment shall be properly assessed by qualified individuals and appropriate services shall be rendered within the defined capability of the hospital.

Individuals shall be accorded impartial access to treatment or accommodations that are available or medically indicated, regardless of race, creed, sex, national origin, or sources of payment of care.

In the *Guerrero* decision the court noted that:

> If a hospital has been accredited by the Joint Commission on Hospital Accreditation, such Commission requires that its accredited hospital with emergency room facilities render emergency (care) to all who need it. It is arguable that by asking for and receiving accreditation, the hospital has undertaken a duty to the public, modifying the common law.

These decisions seem to suggest that if there is a reasonable basis for suspecting that emergency care is necessary, a patient has a right to be examined and treated by a physician if the patient gets to the hospital emergency room.

The Emergency Transfer

It has also been legally established that a hospital's obligation to provide care continues even after the emergency condition has been stabilized until the patient is properly transferred or is medically fit for discharge (*Methodist Hospital v. Ball*, 1961). More recent decisions suggest that courts are likely to continue their view that public policy requires that emergency care be provided to those who need it (*Thompson v. Sun City Community Hospital*, 1984; *St. Joseph's Hospital v. Maricopa Co.*, 1984). In *Thompson* the Arizona Supreme Court found the hospital liable for transferring a patient to the county hospital solely on economic grounds (Curran, 1985).

Although hospitals are within their legal rights to stabilize emergency patients and transfer them to other hospitals, they must do so in a non-negligent and reasonable manner. A Louisiana Court addressed the "reasonableness" issue in *Joyner v. Alton Ochsner Medical Foundation* (1970) and ruled in favor of the hospital. In *Joyner* after providing initial emergency treatment, the hospital refused to admit the patient without a deposit and transferred him. The patient sued for pain and suffering incurred during the transfer.

Conversely, in *Jones v. City of New York Hospital for Joint Diseases* (1954), the New York Supreme Court found the hospital liable for transferring a patient without rendering emergency surgery. In a recent case, a Pennsylvania Supreme Court in *Riddle Memorial Hospital v. Dohan* (1984), reaffirmed the lower court's decision that the hospital had acted reasonable in allowing the patient to be transferred. An interesting aspect of this case was that the patient's private physician was the attending physician at Riddle and favored the transfer to another hospital.

Despite the present legal standards requiring hospitals to provide emergency care to those who need it, the increased emphasis on cost containment is transforming medical care from a social good to an economic one. Not only has the rise of for-profit hospitals challenged the traditional social commitment of hospitals to provide emergency services to the uninsured and poor, but so has the lessening of the social commitment on the part of government itself. The government's emphasis on cost containment has made quality of care and equity of access concerns secondary issues (Greensberg, 1984). This new economics of medicine means a fierce competition among hospitals that must keep one eye on healing and the other on the bottom line. Providing hospital care to the medically indigent and the poor has become an intolerable expense on the part of many hospitals.

In fact, some hospitals have closed completely or have chosen not to provide emergency care because of the financial situation created by medically indigent. In Los Angeles the problem of uncompensated care was a contributing factor in the closing of 11 hospitals since 1985 (Brider, 1987). Several other hospitals have chosen to discontinue their participation in the Los Angeles area's trauma network because of the increasing number of uninsured trauma patients (Brider, 1987). Other hospitals have downgraded their emergency rooms to avoid having to accept uninsured emergency trauma cases (Brom, 1986). These situations coupled with the nationwide increase in the closures of private for-profit hospitals and public hospitals in the inner city (Rice, 1987) are making it increasingly difficult for the medically indigent to locate a source of hospital care.

PUBLIC POLICY RESPONSE TO DUMPING

Texas became the first state to effect comprehensive regulations that specifically deal with the dumping problem (Smith, 1986). The regulations which are mandated by Texas law and were promulgated by the Texas State Board of Health (Ellis, 1985) became effective in April, 1986. The regulations prohibit dumping of emergency patients and ensure that patients are transferred only with their informed consent (when possible) and for valid medical reasons (Relman, 1986). The regulations also require hospitals to submit a transfer policy to the Texas Department of Health. Hospitals not submitting an acceptable policy by a specified time risk losing their license to operate and fines of not more than 1,000 dollars for each violation (Smith, 1986). The legislation was prompted by Parkland Memorial Hospital in Dallas which effectuated a policy and study of patient transfers in 1983 (Reed, Cawley, and Anderson, 1986).

In 1983 the Texas legislature enacted a law making hospitals and physicians liable to felony prosecutions if they deny medical care to individuals because of socioeconomic considerations. At the time of the legislation, Texas ranked 48th among the states in the level of payments to hospitals for the poor. In 1983 New York passed a statute that makes economic emergency refusals a misdemeanor punishable by a fine of $1,000 and a year in jail for the hospital personnel involved. The State of New York may also revoke a hospital's operating license for denying emergency care after a judicial hearing. In June 1985 South Carolina enacted an anti-dumping law which included a civil penalty of up to $10,000 if violated by a hospital (Dallek and Waxman, 1986).

Some 25 states have enacted legislation requiring hospitals to provide emergency care regardless of ability to pay and requiring that patients be stabilized before transfer (Ansell and Schiff, 1987). However, many of the state statutes are ineffective and are rarely enforced. Treiger (1986:1186) notes that "the central weakness of most state statutes is that they do not contain a clear definition of emergency services" and those states that have remedies, have weak ones. For example, in Georgia and South Carolina fines range from 100 to 500 dollars (Treiger, 1986). At the local government level in 1986, Alameda County and Los Angeles County California have developed a set of guidelines for hospital transfers.

At the federal level, the Consolidated Omnibus Budget Reconciliation Act (COBRA) enacted by Congress in 1985 (Public Law 99-272) prohibits patient dumping. The law requires hospitals to provide a medical examination and the necessary treatment to stabilize the condition of anyone who comes to the hospital with severe, acute symptoms (Bishop, 1987; Parks and Dallek, 1986). A hospital or physician found in violation of this requirement is subject to a civil penalty of up to $25,000 per case. Brookside Hospital, a public hospital in San Pablo, California, became the first facility to face fines and sanctions under the law. The U.S. Department of Health and Human Services (DHHS) began investigating five cases of alleged patient dumping at the hospital (Bishop, 1987). If found in violation, the hospital would not only be subject to civil penalty as its prescribed by law but also could be denied its Medicare/Medicaid reimbursements which in 1986 amounted to nearly $25 million (Bishop, 1987). The legislation also requires that if an emergency exists, a hospital must stabilize the patient or transfer him/her to a facility that can; a hospital cannot transfer an unstable patient unless another facility can offer better treatment (Burda, 1987).

By late 1987 DHHS had received only 33 complaints of patient dumping. Table 1 provides a listing of complaints filed with DHHS as of October, 1987. More than 50 percent of the complaints came from the State of Texas. Only five actions had been taken against hospitals (Burda, 1987). The University of Chicago Hospital was charged with dumping a gunshot victim in July 1987. DHHS issued termination of Medicare participation against the hospital. After adding a trauma team and promising such an incident would not occur again the facility was exonerated (Burda, 1987). By January 31, 1988 DHHS had received 129 complaints and fines had been levied and Medicare termination disqualification had been initiated against only two hospitals. By mid-1988 DHHS had received 188 complaints alleging patient dumping and 53 were found not to have complied with the law (Tolchin, 1988). By late 1988, 61 hospitals were found by DHHS to have violated the anti-dumping law (Ansberry, 1988).

Despite the increase in anti-dumping legislation at the state and federal government levels, several shortcomings have become evident and need to be addressed. First, legislation needs to provide mechanisms for monitoring and enforcement/compliance. Second, legislation needs to more clearly and precisely define what a medical emergency is and what it means to stabilize a person before

TABLE 1. Hospital Dumping Complaints Filed with DHHS*

Region	Date Complaint Received	Name of Hospital	Section of COBRA Alleged Noncompliant	In Progress	In Compliance	Out of Compliance
III	01/16/87	Mary Washington Fredericksburg, VA	Treatment and transfer for active labor	X		
IV	04/27/87	Methodist, Somerville IN	Stabilizing treatment, transfer	X		
	12/04/87	Jennie Stuart Hopkinsville, KY	Stabilizing treatment, transfer	X		
	01/08/87	Marymount, London, KY	Stabilizing treatment		X	
	01/27/87	George County/Mobile Lucedale, MS	Treatment, transfer for active labor		X	
	02/24/87	Goodlark, Dickson, TN	Stabilizing treatment		X	
	04/08/87	Jackson-Madison, Jackson, TN	Stabilizing treatment	X		
	04/01/87	Methodist Evangelical Louisville, KY	Treatment, transfer	X		
VI	01/05/87	Humana, Clear Lake, TX	Stabilizing treatment, transfer	X		
	01/06/87	Dermot-Chicot Dermot, TX	Screening, treatment, transfer active labor	X		
	04/08/87	South Plains Amherst, TX	Treatment, transfer	X		
	05/05/87	Fannin County, Bonham, TX	Treatment, transfer	X		

TABLE 1 (continued)

Region	Date Complaint Received	Name of Hospital	Section of COBRA Alleged Noncompliant	In Progress	In Compliance	Out of Compliance
	05/05/87	Lillian, Sonora, TX	Treatment, transfer	X		
	05/05/87	Wintergarden Memorial Dilly, TX	Treatment, transfer	X		
	05/05/87	Charter Community Cleveland, TX	Treatment, transfer		(termination underway)	X
	05/12/87	Trinity Memorial Trinity, TX	Treatment, transfer	X		
	05/12/87	Riverside Corpus Christi, TX	Treatment, transfer	X		
	05/12/87	Terrell Community Terrell, TX	Treatment, transfer	X		
	05/12/87	San Saba, San Saba, TX	Treatment, transfer	X		
	05/12/87	Mitchell County Colorado City, TX	Treatment, transfer	X		
	05/12/87	South Arlington Medical Center, Arlington, TX	Treatment, transfer	X		
	05/27/87	Oakgrove Louisiana West Carroll Parish, LA	Treatment, transfer	X		
	05/27/87	Central Texas Memorial Center, Hearne, TX	Treatment, transfer	X		
	04/15/87	Trinity Memorial Trinity, TX	Treatment, transfer	X		

Region	Date Complaint Received	Name of Hospital	Section of COBRA Alleged Noncompliant	In Progress	In Compliance	Out of Compliance
	12/30/86	Lewisville Medical Lewisville, TX	Treatment	X		
	01/28/87	McAllen Medical McAllen, TX	Refuse to accept indigent transfers		X	
	02/17/87	Detar, Victoria, TX	Treatment, transfer for active labor	X		
	02/20/87	Alvin Community Alvin, TX	Treatment, transfer		X	
	11/21/86	HCA Valley Brownsville, TX	Treatment, transfer		X	
	04/01/87	Colonial, Terrell, TX	Treatment, transfer		X	
	04/01/87	Wilson N. Jones Sherman, TX	Screening, treatment, transfer		X	
IX	03/18/87	Brookside, San Pablo, TX	Treatment, transfer		(termination rescinded)	X
	04/09/87	Los Medanos Pittsburg, CA	Transfer	X		

Source: Committee on Government Operations, *Equal Access to Health Care: Patient Dumping*, Hearing Before a Subcommittee on Government Operations, House of Representatives, 100th Congress, 1st Session, July 22, 1987 (Washington, DC: Government Printing Office, 1988), pp. 210-211.

*As of October 9, 1987.

transfer (see Ansell and Schiff, 1987). Defining stabilization is most important because as Relman (1985:373) points out "'stabilization' of emergency cases is a notion used by hospital managers to justify transfers for economic reasons, but it is an elusive and dangerous concept." In other words, present legislation may still allow patient's condition to be misrepresented when a private hospital transfers them to a public hospital.

Third, the legislation needs to more closely address the medical aspects of patient dumping. The point here is that patients in need of emergency care are being denied appropriate care and treatment. Studies (Himmelstein, Woolhandler, and Harnly, 1984; Anderson, Cowley, and Andrulis, 1984; Schiff et al., 1986; and Wren, 1985) have shown, and reports by the popular media have noted (Okie, 1986; "Checking the Patients," 1986, 1987), that transfers have jeopardized the patients' well-being because of delayed treatment or lack of treatment. The transfer also leads to problems in testing the lab procedures duplication (Hicks et al., 1986) and increased pain and suffering on the part of the transferred patients (Ansell and Schiff, 1987).

In response to these concerns the Health Care Financing Administration in DHHS, the agency charged with enforcement, proposed new anti-dumping regulations. Congress adopted the regulations as an amendment to COBRA in April 1986. The regulations become effective on August 1, 1987. The gist of the regulations are: (1) when pregnant patients are in active labor, they cannot be transferred; (2) a hospital cannot transfer a patient unless that person's medical condition has been stabilized; (3) a transfer can take place if a doctor certifies in writing that the transfer to the receiving hospital outweighs the risk of transfer if better treatment is available. The regulations define stabilize as "providing medical treatment of the condition necessary to assure, within reasonable medical probability, that no material deterioration of the condition is likely to result from the transfer" (Robinson, 1987:36). Congress increased the civil monetary penalty from $25,000 to $50,000 (U.S. House of Representatives, 1987).

Despite these changes, the legislation needs to be amended with additional provisions. First, the legislation needs to require that a *memo of transfer* be signed by the sending hospital physician and the receiving hospital physician. This process would serve to first document the transfer through written record and second place accountability on physicians. Second, the legislation needs to require a posted notice in hospitals about the law. Hill-Burton hospitals are required by DHHS to post notices concerning their Hill-Burton obligations (Rice and Jones, 1985). This provision would help make the law more knowledgeable to individuals and would perhaps increase compliance.

CONCLUSION

Hospitals whether public or private (for-profit) exist to serve the needs of patients. Yet present government policy seems to be telling hospitals that they must become more cost conscious–that is, act like competitive businesses. In this kind of climate hospital care for the indigent and the uninsured is not a very high concern particularly for private for-profit hospitals. As Relman (1985:372) observes "[w]hen business considerations dominate the behavior of hospital management, the poor will be inevitably neglected." Patient dumping may be viewed as a most serious form of neglect.

While public policy is now addressing the patient dumping problem at the federal and state level, more comprehensive laws are needed that require all hospitals, regardless of ownership, to treat all emergency patients who arrive at their doors. Less than half of the states have enacted statutes concerning emergency medical care or health care for those without insurance. If economic rather than medical reasons continue to be the motivation for patient dumping for hospitals not to provide care, then individuals will continue to be at high risk of not receiving necessary hospital care. This will be especially the case for the black community.

NOTES

1. The four largest private profit-making hospital chains, Hospital Corporation of America, Humana, Inc., American Medical International and National Medical Enterprises, earned 297 million, 193 million, 155 million, and 127 million dollars, respectively, in 1984 (Kraft, 1985).

2. The largest percentage of the total uninsured are found in the West South Central and Mountain geographical regions in the U.S. with 20.2 percent and 19.2 percent, respectively. The New England and Middle Atlantic regions have the smallest percentage of the total uninsured with 10.5 percent and 12.5 percent, respectively (Sulvetta and Swartz, 1986).

3. About 23 million low income individuals were covered by Medicaid in fiscal year 1986 (Treiger, 1986, note 18).

4. Some 29 million aged and 3 million disabled individuals are covered under Medicare (Treiger, 1986, note 18).

5. A similar ruling applicable to doctors can be traced to the Indiana Supreme Court in *Hurley v. Eddingfield* (1901).

6. Unlike nonfeasance, malfeasance is an affirmative act causing injury or increased risk of harm to another. Malfeasance imposes a duty to provide aid.

7. A Georgia Court of Appeals has ruled that a public hospital that maintains emergency facilities open to the general public cannot arbitrarily refuse to provide emergency services to any member of the public in need of such services (see *Williams v. Hospital Authority of Hall Co.* [1969].

REFERENCES

Aaron, H. J. (1984). "Prospective Payment: The Next Disappointment?" *Health Affairs* (Fall): 102-107.

Americans at Risk: The Case of the Medically Uninsured. Hearings Before the Senate Special Committee on Aging (1985). 99th Congress, 1st Session.

Anderson, R. J., Cowley, K. A. and Andrulis, D. P. (1984). "The Evolution of A Public Hospital Transfer Policy." Paper presented at the 112th Annual Meeting of the American Public Health Association. Anaheim, CA, November 13.

Annas, G. J. (1986). "Your Money or Your Life: 'Dumping' Uninsured Patients from Hospital Emergency Wards." *American Journal of Public Health* (January):74-77.

Ansberry, C. (1988). "Dumping the Poor: Despite Federal Law, Hospitals Still Reject Sick Who Can't Pay." *Wall Street Journal* (November 29): A1, A10.

Ansell, D. A. and Schiff, R. L. (1987). "Patient Dumping: Status, Implications and Policy Recommendations." *Journal of the American Medical Association* 257 (March 20): 1500-1502.

Baldwin, M. F. (1985). "Lawmakers Focus on Hospital DRG Squeeze." *Modern Health Care* (March): 54-58.

Berg, T. (1983). "Major Corporations Ask Workers to Pay More of Health Care." *The New York Times* (September 12): A1.

Bishop, Katherine (1987). "Hospital May Lose Funds Over Transfers of Poor." *The New York Times* (April 1).

Bovbjerg, R. R. and Kopit, W. G. (1986). "Coverage and Care for the Medically Indigent: Public and Private Options." *Indiana Law Review* 19:857-917.

Brider, P. (1987). "Too Poor To Pay: The Scandal of Patient Dumping." *American Journal of Nursing* (November): 1447-1449.

Brom, T. (1986). "Death By a Thousand Cuts." *California Lawyer* 6 (April): 19-20.

Burda, D. (1987). "Dumping Law Spurs Look at E D Risk Management." *Hospitals* (July 20): 34-38.

"Checking the Patients Before His Credit." (Editorial) (1986). *The Atlanta Constitution* (April 1): A-14.

Comment (1974). "Liability of Private Hospital Emergency Rooms for Refusal to Provide Emergency Care." *Mississippi Law Journal* 45:1003-1028.

Curran, W. J. (1985). "Law-Medicine Notes: Economic and Legal Considerations in Emergency Care." *New England Journal of Medicine* (February 7) :374-375.

Dallek, G. and Waxman, J. (1986). "Patient Dumping: A Crisis in Emergency Medical Care for the Indigent." *Clearinghouse Review* (April): 1413-1417.

Dowell, Michael A. (1984). "Indigent Access to Hospital Emergency Room Services." *Clearinghouse Review* (October 1984): 483-492.

Duncan, R. P. and Vogel, W. B. (1988). "Uncompensated Care and the Inpatient Transfer." Presented at the Annual Meeting of the American Public Health Association. Boston, MA.

Editorial (1982). "Hospitals Said 'No.'" *Des Moines Tribune* (May 18).

Ellis, Virginia (1985). "Compromise Paves Way for Outlining 'Patient Dumping.'" *Dallas Times Herald* (December 13).

Fine, J. E. (1983). *Journal of Urban and Contemporary Law* 24:123-149.

Frank, C. (1985). "Dumping the Poor: Private Hospitals Risk Suits." *American Bar Association Journal* 71 (March): 25.

Friedman, E. (1982). "Special Report–The Dumping Dilemma: Finding What's Fair." *Hospitals* (September 18):75-84.

General Accounting Office (1985), *Medicare: PPS Impact on Post-Hospital Long Term Care Services* (Washington, DC: GAO/PEMO-85-8, February 21).

Greensberg, D.S. (1984). "Health Care Thrift Spurs Patient Dumping." *Los Angeles Times* (November 12).

Hicks, T. C., Danzl, D. F., Thomas, D. M., and Flint, L. M. (1986). "Resuscitation and Transfer of Trauma Patients: A Prospective Study." *Annals of Emergency Medicine*, 296-299.

Himmelstein, D. U., Woolhandler, S. and Harnly, M. (1984). "Patient Transfers: Medical Practice as Social Triage." *American Journal of Public Health* 74:494-497.

"Hospitals in Cost Squeeze 'Dump' More Patients Who Can't Pay Bills" (1985). *Wall Street Journal* (March 8).

Inglehart, J.K. (1985). "Medical Care of the Poor: A Growing Problem." *New England Journal of Medicine* (January):59-63.

Joint Commission on the Accreditation of Hospitals (1984). *Accreditation Manual of Hospitals*, 1985 ed: (Chicago: Joint Commission on the Accreditation of Hospitals).

Klaidman, D. (1986). "D.C. General: Hospital or Dumping Ground?" *The Washington Post* (December 29).

Kraft, J. (1985). "Hospitals for Profit: What Price Care?" *Los Angeles Times* (March 31): 1,33.

Marsh, Barbara (1988). "The Medical Indigence Crisis." *Crain's Chicago Business* 11(43) (October 24):1, 100-104.

McCormick, B. (1986). "15% of Transfers Seen as 'Dumping.'" *Hospitals* (October 5):146.

Millenson, M. (1987). "The Unhealthy Medical Care of the Poor." *Business and Society Review* (Spring): 40-43.

Milligan, C. J., Jr. (1986). "Provisions of Uncompensated Care in American Hospitals: The Role of Tax Code, The Federal Courts, Catholic Health Care Facilities, and Local Governments in Defining the Problem of Access for the Poor." *Catholic Lawyer* 31(1): 7-34.

Morrisey, M. A., Sloan, F. A., and Valvona, J. (1988a). "Post Hospitals Transfers Under Medicare Prospective Payment." *Health Affairs*. (In Press).

Morrisey, M. A., Sloan, F. A., and Valvona, J. (1988b). "Medicare Prospective Payment and Posthospital Transfers to Subacute Care." *Medical Care* 26(7) (July): 685-698.

Mueller, K. J. and Comer, J. C. (1987). "Providers' Predictions of Effects of the Prospective Payment System." *Journal of Health and Human Resources Administration* (Fall 1987): 147-155.

Okie, S. (1986). "'Dumping' Patients into Public Hospitals May Shorten Lives, Study Says." *The Washington Post* (February 27):A-14.

Parks, M. C. and Dallek, G. (1986). "New COBRA Legislation Adopts Many Changes in Medicare and Other Health Programs." *Clearinghouse Review* (August/September): 562-572.

Pfeiffer, D. and Christian, P. (1987). "Impact of the Federal Prospective Payment System Upon Long-Term Care Related Medicare Patients." *Journal of Health and Human Resources Administration* (Fall): 115-146.

Reed, W. G., Cawley, K. A. and Anderson, R. J. (1986). "Special Report: The Effect of a Public Hospital's Transfer Policy on Patient Care." *New England Journal of Medicine* (November 27):1428-1432.

Reinhardt, Ewe (1985). "Editorial: Health and Hot Potatoes." *The Washington Post* (March 16):2.

Relman, A. S. (1985): "Economic Considerations In Emergency Care: What are Hospitals For?" *New England Journal of Medicine* (February 7): 372.373.

Relman, A. S. (1986). "Texas Eliminates Dumping: A Start Toward Equity in Hospital Care." *New England Journal of Medicine* (February 27): 578-579.

Rice, M. F. (1985/86). "The Urban Public Hospital: Its Importance to the Black Community." *Urban League Review* 9(2) (Winter): 64-70.

Rice, M. F. (1987). "Inner-City Hospital Closures/Relocations: Race, Income Status and Legal Issues." *Social Science and Medicine* 24(11): 889-896.

Rice, M. F. and Jones, W., Jr. (1985). "Public Policy and Black Health Care: A Civil Rights Perspective." In *Institutional Racism and Black America* edited by Mfanya D. Tryman. (Lexington, MA: Ginn Press): 67-99.

Robinson, M. L. (1987). "Patient 'Dumping' Regulations Offer Little Guidance." *Hospitals* (September 5):35-36.

Rowland, D. and Davis, K. (1982). "The Uninsured and Inpatient Hospital Care." Paper Presentation at the 110th Annual Meeting of the American Public Association Annual Meeting. Montreal, Canada, November.

Sager, A. (1983). "The Reconfiguration of Urban Hospital Care." In *Cities and Sickness: Health Care in Urban America* edited by Ann L. Green and Scott Green. (Beverly Hills: Sage Publications).

Schiff, R. L., Ansell, D. A., Schlosser, J. E., Idris, A. H., Morrison, A. and Whitman, S. (1986). "Transfers to a Public Hospital: A Prospective Study of 467 Patients." *New England Journal of Medicine* (February 27):552-557.

Smith. (1986). TDH Rules on Hospital Transfers Take Effect April 1" *Texas Medicine* 82 (March): 59-62.

Sulvetta, M. B. and Swartz, K. (1986). *The Uninsured and Uncompensated Care: A Chartbook* (Washington, DC: National Health Policy Forum).

Tolchin, M. (1988). "U.S. Seeks to Require Treatment of All Hospital Emergency Cases." *The New York Times* (June 18): 1, 8.

Trafford, A., Dworkin, P., Carey, J., and McAuliffe, K. (1986). "The New World of Health Care." *U.S. News and World Report* (April 14): 60-63.

Treiger, K. I. (1986). "Preventing Patient Dumping: Sharpening the COBRA's Fangs." *New York University Law Review* 61 (December): 1186-1223.

U.S. House of Representatives (1987). *Omnibus Budget Reconciliation Act of 1987: Conference Report to Accompany H.R. 3545* (Washington, DC: Government Printing Office, December 21, 1987).

Valda, M. I. (1983). "The Financial Impact of Prospective Payment on Hospitals" *Health Affairs* (Spring): 112-119.

Wehr, B. (1982). "Hospitals, Insurers, Patients Feeling Pinch of Federal Cutbacks in Medicare, Medicaid Funds." *Congressional Quarterly Weekly Report* (July 17).

Wing, K. R. and Campbell, J. R. (1985). "The Emergency Room Admission: How Far Does the 'Open Door' Go?" *University of Detroit Law Review* 63:119-144.

Wren, K. (1985). "Sounding Board: No Insurance, No Admission." *New England Journal of Medicine* (February 7): 373-374.

COURT CASES

Birmingham Baptist Hospital v. Crews, 157 Ala. So. 224 (1934).
Fjerstad v. Knutson, 271 N.W. 2d 8 (S.D. 1978).
Guerrero v. Copper Queen Hospital, 112 Ariz. 104,537 P.2d 1329 (1975).
Harper v. Baptist Medical Center-Princeton, 341 So. 2d 133 (Ala. 1976).
Hill v. Ohio County, 468 S.W. 2d 306 (Ky. 1971).
Hunt v. Palm Springs General Hospital, 352 So. 2d 582 (Fla. 1977).
Hurley v. Eddingfield, 156 Ind. 416, 59 N.E. 1058 (1901).

Jones v. City of New York Hospital for Joint Diseases, 134 N.Y.S. 2d 779 (Supt.Ct. 1954).

Joyner v. Alton Ochsner Medical Foundation, 230 So. 2d 913 (La.Ct.App. 1970).

LeJeune Road Hospital Inc. v. Watson, 171 So. 2d 202 (Fla.Dist.Ct.App. 1965).

Mercy Medical Center v. Winnebago Co., 206 N.W. 2d 198 (Wisc. 1973).

Methodist Hospital v. Ball, 50 Tenn. App. 460, 362 S.W. 2d 475 (1961).

New Biloxi Hospital Inc. v. Frazier, 146 Miss. So. 2d (1962).

O'Neill v. Montefiore Hospital, 202 N.Y.S. 2d 436 (1960).

Riddle Memorial Hospital v. Dohan, 504 Pa. 571, 471 A. 2d 1314 (1984).

St. Joseph's Hospital v. Maricopa Co., 688 Ariz. P.2d 986 (1984).

Thompson v. Sun City Community Hospital, 688 Ariz. P.2d 605 (1984).

Williams v. Hospital Authority of Hall County, 168 Se. 2d 336 (Court of Appeals of Georgia, Division No. 3, 1969).

Wilmington General Hospital v. Manlove, 54 Del. 15, 174 A.2d 135 (1961).

Chapter 3

Determinants of Health Services Utilization Among the Black and White Elderly

Verna M. Keith
Woodrow Jones

SUMMARY. Andersen's behavioral model was used to assess whether factors predictive of health services utilization are the same or different for elderly blacks and whites. We hypothesized that because the black elderly have fewer resources, lower psychological well-being, and are in worse health, situational and attitudinal factors suggested by the model have different effects for blacks and whites. Using three measures of utilization–physician contact, hospital contact, and nights hospitalized–our findings show some support for differential effects, particularly in the case of physician contact. Neither resource factors such as health insurance nor psychological well-being were predictive of utilization within the black population. We conclude with some suggestions for future research.

Use of health care services by the elderly is a topic of increasing concern in the United States."[1] Escalating health care cost, disproportionate use of services by the elderly, and the increasing number of individuals aged 65 and over form the basis for this concern.[2] Over the past few years, a number of studies have examined why

Time for the first author to complete this project was supported by a grant from the National Institute on Aging (RO1-AG06618-01). The authors wish to thank Steve Ellis for computer assistance.

This chapter was originally published in *Journal of Health & Social Policy*, Vol. 1(3) 1990.

and how the elderly use health services.[3] However, few have focused on racial and ethnic differences. Although Jackson[4] first argued some twenty years ago that social inequality based on race and ethnicity affect the aging experience, the area of minority aging remains underdeveloped. If the effects of race and ethnic group membership persist into old age, assumptions of similar determinants of illness behavior in majority and minority elderly are misleading. Moreover, policies which result from such assumptions may not be adequate in meeting the health care needs of the minority elderly. We address these issues by assessing whether various situational and attitudinal determinants of health care utilization are similar for elderly blacks and whites.

Aging, Minorities, and the Use of Health Services

Health services researchers have always been interested in the utilization patterns of various segments of the population, but only recently has there been any focus on the elderly. Research over the past decade has demonstrated that the elderly are prone to be heavy users of medical services.[5] While the elderly represent 11.3 percent of the population, they occupy one-third of all hospital beds and account for approximately one-fourth of all health care expenditures.[6] The number of physician visits per person per year is 8.1 for the population aged 65 and over compared to 6.4 for the general population.[7] Population projections indicate that the number and proportion of elderly will increase well into the next century. If, as policy makers expect, the increasing number of elderly is accompanied by increasing use of physician and hospital services, the health care system will be severely strained.[8] To ensure that adequate health care is available to the aged, and to identify points of appropriate policy intervention, more information is needed on which factors are most influential in determining utilization among the elderly.

Various approaches have been used to explain utilization behavior. Generally these approaches place emphasis on either situational attributes such as socioeconomic status and demographic characteristics, attitudes and beliefs of the user, or organizational aspects of the health care system such as type of service provider.[9] Increasingly, researchers are developing and using more complex models which incorporate situational, attitudinal, and organizational components to explain utilization.[10] The applications of complex models and multivariate statistical techniques have underscored the need to take into account numerous factors, particularly the psychological dimensions of illness. Results from such studies show that, although utilization varies by race/ethnicity, sex, availability of health insurance, and having a regular source of care, self-evaluated health status is particularly influential.[11] Among the elderly, self-rated health status has even stronger explanatory significance than in the general population.[12] However, the extent to which such findings hold for blacks and other minority elderly remains unclear.

With few exceptions, studies of utilization which have included aged blacks and other minority elderly have usually grouped them into one category designated as "nonwhite,"[13] or have been based on samples not representative of the United States: elderly from low income areas.[14] Multivariate analyses using more complex models rarely test for interaction between race and other explanatory variables. Consequently, questions of whether blacks and other minority elderly use health services for the same reasons as whites or whether variables have the same significance for minorities have not been given sufficient attention.

Compared to aged whites, black and other minority elderly are more likely to experience economic hardship,[15] to perceive their health as being poor[16] and, in some studies, to have lower life satisfaction.[17] Over the life course, older blacks in particular have suffered from direct and indirect institutionalized discrimination.[18] Given these disadvantages, it is reasonable to assume that factors such as economic status, health insurance coverage, perceived health status, and psychological well-being may be relatively more influential in explaining utilization patterns for blacks than for whites. Indeed, some supporting evidence for differential determinants for blacks and whites is found in Wan's[19] study of elderly living in low income urban areas. Although self-reported health status was the most influential factor in explaining the number of physician visits in both groups, health insurance coverage was significant for blacks but not for whites. This suggests that affordability is more of a problem for blacks than for whites. Other studies of the general population also lend support to the hypothesis that factors affecting response to illness may be somewhat different for blacks and other minorities. Wolinsky,[20] using a sample of rural blacks and whites of all ages, reported significant racial differences in the effects of a number of factors on use of discretionary health care services. Strand and Jones'[21] study of Indochinese refugees also suggested that cultural variation influences utilization. A study of Hispanics in the southwest found that they encountered greater barriers to care than the population as a whole owing to their lower socioeconomic status and lack of health insurance.[22] Hence, we might expect situational and attitudinal variables to yield different results for blacks and whites.

The Conceptual Model

This study uses the behavioral model developed by Andersen[23] as a guiding framework for examining use of health services among the black and white elderly. The model is the most widely used approach in health services research,[24] and has been used in studies of the elderly.[25] It provides the advantages of identifying groups at risk of encountering barriers to care and of identifying determinants (e.g., insurance) which can be modified through policy intervention.

The behavioral model views use of services as being dependent on three sets of characteristics–predisposing, enabling, and need. Andersen's argument is that individuals with different demographic characteristics (e.g., age, sex, family size, and marital status), social-structural characteristics (e.g., education, occupation, and race), and health beliefs (e.g., locus of control and medical knowledge) have greater or lesser propensity to use services and are therefore "predisposed" to use services at different rates. Individuals with different demographic characteristics also have differing types and amounts of illness. Furthermore, placement in the social structure leads to different life styles and, therefore, to different patterns of utilization. Patterns of use may also vary with the salience of health beliefs.

Enabling characteristics refer to family and community resources which permit the use of services including income, health insurance, and place of residence. Although one may be predisposed to use services, actual use will not occur without sufficient resources and access to health care providers.

Finally, the behavioral model stipulates that individuals must perceive some need for using health services and posits need as the most direct determinant of utilization. Need is measured by self-reports of symptoms, mental well-being, functional limitations, and perceived health status. Thus, the behavioral model incorporates indicators of objective social position, possession of sufficient resources, and subjective evaluation of the need for care. Distribution on these factors are known to differ by race and ethnicity. In multivariate analyses, these differences are often recognized by treating race and ethnicity as one of several predisposing characteristics. Consequently, race becomes one of many independent variables, and little is known about whether blacks and whites are similarly influenced by other model variables nor whether the model explains similar amounts of variance in both groups. In other words, most research using the behavioral model assumes additive effects and the possibility of interaction effects is overlooked.

In this study we address some of the methodological and substantive issues raised in the area of race and utilization. The analysis focuses on two questions: (1) Which factors are more important in determining health services utilization within the two groups? (2) How well does the behavioral model explain utilization by blacks and whites? The answers to these questions should indicate whether additive models are appropriate in studies of health care service use by the elderly, permit identification of groups that encounter barriers to care, and identify factors which may need a policy response to ensure that the elderly have adequate access to services.

DATA AND METHODS

The data for this study were drawn from the 1975 National Survey of the Aged, a probability sample of noninstitutionalized persons aged 65 and older. The survey, one of the few to include enough blacks for separate analysis, attempted to describe the social support, employment, assets, and general living conditions of 2,143 older Americans. Included in the weighted sample were 1,969 whites, 416 blacks, and 31 elderly from other racial and ethnic groups. We excluded the "other" category due to the small number of cases. Bedridden elderly were also excluded because information gathered for this group did not include many variables of interest to the analysis. The resulting sample sizes were 1,505 whites and 397 blacks.

Coding and measurement of all variables appear in the Appendix. The health service measures used in this study are consistent with those used in other utilization studies. Andersen[26] suggests a distinction between contact or exposure (whether an individual visits a health care professional) and volume (how many visits) within a specific time frame. Consequently, physician and hospital contact measures were constructed to indicate exposure to health service in the preceding 12 months. Number of nights hospitalized in the past 12 months will serve as an indicator of hospital volume. Because the number of nights hospitalized is skewed upward by a small percentage of individuals with extended stays, we truncated this variable at 15 or more nights of the 95th percentile.[27] Unfortunately, there is no measure of the number of physician visits.

Need for health care services includes three attitudinal measures (perceived health status, an index of morale, and a measure of loneliness) and one measure of functional health status (the Index of Functional Incapacity). Self-perceived health is used as a general measure of health status. Morale and loneliness are included as measures of need because the elderly with poor psychological well-being may express their condition in terms of physical symptoms. Morale is measured by an additive index composed of six items indicating the elderly's general outlook on life and their surroundings. Loneliness is a single item measure which asks the elderly to assess the degree to which they feel lonely. The Index of Incapacity is an additive index designed to measure the extent to which the elderly are affected by various physical disabilities and able to perform various tasks.

Consistent with other studies using the behavioral model, income, place of residence, and private health insurance are used as indicators of enabling characteristics. Although most elderly in the sample had Medicare or Medicaid, private health insurance was far from universal. Having private health insurance as a supplement to public insurance is associated with higher utilization. Predisposing characteristics include age, sex, education, marital status, living alone as a surrogate for family size, and labor force participation.

Ordinary least squares regression (OLS) is used in the analysis. While two of our utilization measures are dichotomous, we selected OLS over logistic regression for several reasons. First, parameter estimates obtained from OLS are interpreted more easily than those from logistic regression. Second, studies have indicated that when the dependent dichotomy ranges between .25 and .75, estimates are fairly reliable.[28] In addition, Gilbert[29] and Cleary and Angel[30] have reported that a range of .10 to .90 is probably safe. As suggested by Jackson,[31] we estimate separate models for blacks and whites. Such an analytical procedure assists in isolating differential patterns of utilization and in detecting possible interaction effects.

RESULTS

Table 1 presents the means and standard deviations for all variables used in the analysis and permits us to examine initial (zero-order) differences between blacks and whites on each of the independent and dependent variables. Comparisons indicate that the two groups are quite similar on several of the predisposing characteristics–age and living alone. Blacks are slightly more likely to be female, to be widowed, and have lower educational attainment. Labor force participation was slightly higher for whites than for blacks. Although there are no substantial racial differences in place of residence, whites have a definite advantage in terms of income and health insurance.

Racial differences in need for medical care are clearly evident. Blacks do not score as high as whites on the index of general morale and are more likely to be lonely. While these differences are not as large as we might expect, they do suggest that the black elderly have a more negative outlook on life than their white counterparts. Consistent with national estimates,[32] blacks are more likely to rate their health as being poor rather than good or excellent, and show evidence of greater disability as indicated by the index of incapacity. The means presented in the table are based on responses which show that 31 percent of blacks and 13 percent of whites rate

TABLE 1. Means and Standard Deviations for all Variables by Race

	Blacks (N=397)		Whites (N=1,505)	
	Mean	SD	Mean	SD
Predisposing				
Age	72.70	6.40	72.87	6.25
Sex (F)	.62	.49	.59	.49
Education	2.75	1.36	3.81	1.62
Widowed	.48	.50	.36	.48
Living Alone	.33	.47	.32	.47
Labor Force Participation	.13	.34	.15	.37
Enabling				
Income	3420.24	2622.03	6597.07	7738.62
Place of Residence	4.71	1.48	4.09	1.60
Private Health Insurance	.29	.46	.69	.46
Need				
Morale	11.03	2.62	13.07	2.77
Loneliness	2.01	1.00	1.90	.97
Health Status	2.05	.80	1.64	.74
Index of Incapacity	1.81	5.29	.83	1.64
Utilization Measures				
Physician Contact	.81	.39	.81	.39
Hospital Contact	.20	.40	.18	.38
Nights Hospitalized	10.21	4.67	9.50	4.65

[a]Higher scores indicate poorer health.

their health as poor–a substantial difference. Thus, blacks, relative to whites, appear to have greater need for medical treatment and fewer resources for securing care (e.g., lower income and health insurance).

Finally, racial differences in utilization behaviors support common conceptions about inequality in access. Blacks and whites are equally likely to see a physician even though the former perceive their health as being worse and have a more negative outlook on life. Blacks are slightly more likely to be hospitalized and to have slightly longer stays than whites. These differences are not as great as might be expected given that blacks are in worse health and have more disability. The slightly longer stays for blacks do support common perceptions that, due to lack of resources, minorities tend to delay treatment until illness is at a more advanced stage.

The above description provides basic data on model variables. To assess the more complicated questions concerning the effects of predisposing, enabling, and need characteristics on utilization we use regression procedures. Table 2 presents the unstandardized regression coefficients and the explained variance (R^2). Unstandardized coefficients are appropriate for making comparisons across groups. To save space we do not present the standardized coefficients.

Looking first at whether respondents had a physician contact, the data indicate that explanatory variables differ for blacks and whites, supporting the contention of differential effects. Among elderly blacks, being widowed, living alone, being in the labor force, place of residence, and perceived health status are significantly related to whether a physician was visited within the past year. Sex, education, living alone, having private health insurance, and perceived health status affects the probability that whites see a physician. Only two variables, living alone and perceived health status, are significant for both blacks and whites. For whites, both the standardized (not shown) and unstandardized coefficients show that perceived health status is clearly more influential than all other variables in determining a physician visit. Among blacks, however, there is little difference in the importance of labor force participation and perceived health status. Contrary to our hypothesis, morale, loneliness, and resource factors other than employment are not significant for the black elderly.

With the exception of perceived health status, none of the predisposing, enabling, and need variables have a significant effect on whether elderly blacks are hospitalized. Among whites, private health insurance, health status, and functional incapacity are significant. However, the coefficient for health status is considerably larger than the other two. The magnitude of the coefficients also indicates that health status has a greater impact in determining hospitalization among whites than among blacks. Again these findings appear to support the contention of differential effects.

TABLE 2. Regression and R^2 Coefficients for the Effects of Predisposing, Enabling, and Need Characteristics on Health Service Utilization by Black and White Elderly

	Physician	Contact	Hospital	Contact	Nights Hospitalized	
	Black	White	Black	White	Black	White
Predisposing						
Age	.001	.003	.002	.000	.009	.120**
Sex	.042	.052*	−.052	−.016	1.020	.263
Education	.014	.022**	.019	.011	.733	.232
Widowed	.103*	−.023	.058	−.018	1.227	1.134
Living Alone	−. 092*	−.067*	−.063	−.019	.749	.120
In Labor Force	−.141*	−.053	−.055	−.021	.756	−.272
Enabling						
Income	.000	.000	−.000	.000	.0001	.000
Place of Residence	.003*	.000	.015	−.007	.416	.836
Private Health insurance	.018	.090***	.024	.047*	.844	.620
Need						
Morale	.001	−.004	.003	−.005	.239	−.246*
Loneliness	.014	.019	.031	.018	−.251	−.559
Health Status	.131**	.110**	.059*	.110*	−1.632	.397
Index of Incapacity	.001	.010	.002	.021*	−.031	.369**
R^2	.16	.08	.04	.08	.15	.17

*P<.05
**P<.01
***P<.001

When considering the number of nights hospitalized among those who entered the hospital, none of the variables are significant for blacks. For whites, age, place of residence, morale, and functional incapacity determine number of nights hospitalized with functional incapacity having the largest effect. Thus, for blacks length of stay is unrelated to demographic characteristics, resources, and perceptions. These findings suggest that determinants of the length of stay among hospitalized elderly are different for blacks and whites. However, a note of caution must be observed in assessing these particular findings. In the analysis of nights hospitalized we are dealing with a smaller number of respondents, having eliminated those who were not hospitalized. Hence the number of black respondents are too small to be overly confident.

The next issue addressed is the degree to which the behavioral model explains the use of health services by elderly blacks and whites. Examination of the R^2 coefficients (see Table 2) generally indicate that the model is a poor predictor for both groups with no more than 17 percent of the variance explained on any dependent variable, nights hospitalized for whites. The racial differences in the degree of predictive efficiency depend upon the specific behavior under consideration. For example, the model is more efficient in explaining physician contact among blacks than whites. However, on the remaining utilization measures, the model explains slightly more variance for whites.

DISCUSSION

This study used Andersen's behavioral model to examine whether similar factors predict use of health services by black and white elderly. We hypothesized that because minority elderly are victims of institutionalized discrimination over the life course, predictive factors suggested by the model have different effects for blacks and whites. The findings provide some support for the hypothesis. The probability of seeing a physician differs for various subgroups of elderly whites and blacks, and the characteristics defining these subgroups differ within the two racial groups. We attach particular significance to the findings for physician contact given that physicians act as the primary gatekeepers to the health care system. Few of the model variables, however, significantly affect whether elderly blacks are hospitalized. None are predictive of the number of nights blacks are hospitalized but several are predictive for whites. The findings suggest that factors other than individual characteristics and need for health care determine whether blacks are hospitalized. Among elderly blacks, entering the hospital and length of time hospitalized may be more dependent upon physician discretion and other factors not included in the model.

The behavioral model explained a relatively small proportion of the variance in the use of health services by both blacks and whites. Other researchers have also noted the problem of low explanatory power.[33] One possible explanation for the low predictability of the model is that because physician visits and hospitalization are covered by Medicare and Medicaid, the effects of predisposing and enabling characteristics are no longer important. Snider[34] suggests that the model is more appropriate for explaining the elderly's use of ancillary services such as health maintenance and preventive health care because these services are not covered by insurance. Wolinsky et al.[35] suggest that the poor showing of the model may result from lack of complete specification of its components. For example, community level enabling variables (e.g., physician-population ratio, prevailing charges, etc.) are rarely included in tests of the model but might add a great deal to understanding utilization patterns of both minority and majority elderly. Both Dutton[36] and Kronenfeld[37] have found that delivery system characteristics exert a significant influence on utilization. Aguirre and Bigelow[38] also hypothesize that the relationship between ethnicity or minority group membership and use of health services may depend in part on the specific ethnic or minority group's share of the community's total population and its degree of participation in the delivery system. Unfortunately, the data did not permit us to examine any of these alternatives.

Although we found some support for the usefulness of examining determinants of health services use separately for blacks and whites, further research along these lines is needed. Particularly enlightening would be an analysis of racial differences in the number of physician visits per year, an issue we are not able to address in this study. Future studies should also include utilization measures which tap quality and continuity of care. It is well known that members of minority groups are more likely to use outpatient services rather than private physicians.[39] It is also generally agreed that care by a private physician on a regular basis provides more continuity and, consequently, better quality care. Thus, a more comprehensive understanding of the black elderly's use of health care services requires an evaluation of quality as well as quantity. In addition, future research should build upon suggestions that delivery system characteristics and ethnic participation in the delivery system be added to the behavioral model to improve its explanatory power.

APPENDIX:
Measurement of Utilization, Predisposing, Enabling, and Need Variables

Variables	Measurement	
Utilization		
Physician Contact	1	Yes
	0	No
Hospital Contact	1	Yes
	0	No
Nights Hospitalized	1-15	
Predisposing		
Age	Age in years	
Sex	1	Female
	0	Male
Education	1-7	(None to College graduate or higher)
Widowed	1	Yes
	0	No
Living Alone	1	Yes
	0	No
Labor Force Participation	1	In Labor Force
	0	Not in Labor Force
Enabling		
Income	Total Annual Family Income	
Place of Residence	1-6	(Farm to large metropolitan area)
Private Health Insurance	1	Yes
	0	No

Variables	Measurement
Need	
Morale	Agree, depends, or disagree with 6 items. High morale coded 3.

1. Days are too short for all I want to do.
2. Life of the average person getting worse, not better.
3. Nowadays a person has to live pretty much for today and let tomorrow take care of itself.
4. Can't help feeling that my life is not very useful.
5. Most people lose respect for a man who has retired.
6. Children don't care anything about their parents except for what they can get out of them.

Loneliness	How often do you feel lonely?

1. Never
2. Rarely
3. Sometimes
4. Often

Health Status

1. Good
2. Fair
3. Poor

Index of Incapacity

Ability to perform without restriction (0); ability to perform but with difficulty (1); inability or ability to perform only with assistance (2):

1.   Get out of doors.
2.   Walk up or down stairs.
3.   Get about house.
4.   Take bath.
5.   Dress and put on shoes.
6.   Cut toenails.

REFERENCE NOTES

1. Russell, L., An aging population and the use of medical care. *Medical Care* 19:633-643, 1981; Wan T.T.H. and B.G. Odell, Factors affecting the use of social and health services for the elderly. *Aging and Society* 1:95-115, 1981.

2. Roos, N., E. Shapiro, and L.L. Roos, Aging and the demand for health services: Which aged and whose demand? *The Gerontologists* 24:31-36, 1984; Wolinsky, F.D., D.K. Miller, J. Prendergast, M.J. Creel, and M.N. Chavez, Health services utilization among the noninstitutionalized elderly. *Journal of Health and Social Behavior* 24:325-36, 1983.

3. Wolinsky et al., Health services utilization; Branch, L.G., A. Jette, C. Evashwick, M. Polansky, G. Rowe, and P. Diehr, Toward understanding elders' health services utilization. *Journal of Community Health* 7:80-91, 1981; Eve, S. and H. Friedsam, Multivariate analysis of health care services utilization among older Texans. *Journal of Health and Human Resources Administration* 3:169-191, 1980.

4. Jackson, J.J., Social gerontology and the Negro: A review. *Gerontologist* 7:168-78, 1967.

5. Russell, L., An aging population and the use of medical care.

6. Kart, C., E.S. Metress, and J.F. Metress, *Aging and Health: Biological and Social Perspectives*. Menlo Park, CA: Addison Wesley, 1978.

7. Travino, F. and A. Moss, *Health Indicators for Hispanic, Black, and White Americans*. DHHS Publication 84-1576. Washington DC: U.S. Government Printing Office, 1984.

8. Haug, M., Age and medical care utilization patterns. *Journal of Gerontology* 36:103-11, 1981.

9. McKinlay, J., Some approaches and problems in the study of the use of health services: An overview. *Journal of Health and Social Behavior* 13:115-152, 1972; Shortell, S., Factors associated with the use of health services. In *Introduction to Health Services*, edited by S. Williams and P. Torrens. 2d. ed. New York: Wiley and Sons.

10. Aday, L.A. and R. Andersen, A framework for the study of access to medical care. *Health Services Research* 9:208-20, 1974; Aday, L.A., R. Andersen, and G. Fleming, *Health Care in the U.S.: Equitable for Whom?* Beverly Hills: Sage, 1980.

11. Aday et al., *Health Care in the U.S.*

12. See note 3.

13. Branch et al., Toward understanding elders' health services utilization; Eve, S. and H. Friedsam, Multivariate analysis; Haug, M., Age and medical care.

14. Wan, T.T.H., Use of health services by the elderly in low-income communities. *Milbank Memorial Fund Quarterly* 60:82-107, 1982.

15. Manuel, R. and J. Reid, A comparative demographic profile of the minority and nonminority aged. In *Minority Aging: Sociological and Social Psychological Issues*, edited by R. Manuel. Westport, Conn.: Greenwood Press, 1982, pp. 31-52.

16. Travino, F. and A. Moss, *Health Indicators for Hispanic, Black, and White Americans*.

17. Linn, M.W., K.I. Hunter and P.R. Perry, Differences by sex and ethnicity in the psychological adjustment of the elderly. *Journal of Health and Social Behavior* 20:273-81, 1979.

18. Jackson, J.J., *Minorities and Aging*. Belmont, CA: Wadsworth, 1980.

19. Wan, T.T.H., Use of health services by the elderly.

20. Wolinsky, F.D., Racial differences in illness behavior. *Journal of Community Health* 8:87-101, 1982.

21. Strand, P. and W. Jones, Health service utilization by Indochinese refugees. Paper presented at the annual Southwestern Social Sciences Meeting (San Antonio, Texas), 1981.

22. Andersen, R.S., S. Lewis, A. Giachello, L.A. Aday, and G. Chiu, Access to medical care among the Hispanic population of the Southwestern United States. *Journal of Health and Social Behavior* 22:78-89, 1981.

23. Andersen, R., *Behavioral Model of Families' Use of Health Services*. Research Series No. 25. Chicago: Center for Health Administration Studies, University of Chicago, 1968.

24. Shortell, S., Factors associated with the use of health services.

25. Wan et al., Factors affecting the use of social and health services; Wolinsky et al., Health services utilization; Branch et al., Toward understanding elders' health services utilization.

26. Andersen, R., *Behavioral Model of Families' Use of Health Services*.

27. Wolinsky et al., Health services utilization.

28. Goodman, L., The relationship between modified and usual multiple regression approaches to the analysis of dichotomous variables. In D. Heise (ed.) *Sociological Methodology, 1975*. San Francisco: Jossey-Bass; Knoke, D., A comparison of log-linear and regression models for systems of dichotomous variables. *Sociological Methods and Research* 3:416-34, 1975.

29. Gilbert, N., *Modeling Society*. New York: Macmillan, 1981.

30. Cleary, P. and R. Angel, The analysis of relationships involving a dichotomous dependent variables. *Journal of Health and Social Behavior* 25:334-56, 1984.

31. Jackson, J.J., Some special concerns about race and health: An editorial finale. *Journal of Health and Social Behavior* 16:342, 428-29, 1975.

32. Travino, F. and A. Moss, Health Indicators.

33. Wolinsky et al., Health services utilization; Eve, S. and H. Friedsam, Multivariate analysis.

34. Snider, E.L., Awareness and use of health services by the elderly: A Canadian study. *Medical Care* 18:1177-82, 1980.

35. Wolinsky et al. Health Services Utilization.

36. Dutton, D., Patterns of ambulatory care in five different delivery systems. *Medical Care* 17:221-43, 1979.

37. Kronenfeld, J., Source of ambulatory care and utilization models. *Health Services Research* 15:3-20, 1980.

38. Aguirre, B. and A. Bigelow, The aged in Hispanic groups: A review. *International Journal of Aging and Human Development* 15:35-62, 1983.

39. Wan, T.T.H., Use of health services by the elderly.

Chapter 4

Options for Providing Health Care for the Uninsured: Opportunities for Managed Care

Deborah L. Fritz

SUMMARY. The problem of providing health care for the uninsured has regained national attention. A variety of approaches are being tried across the country including State High Risk Pools and other insurance pools, increased individual policy options, and expansion of Medicaid and Medical Assistance eligibility. One of the key design elements in these approaches is the use of managed care.

A review of important design features and risk factors is presented. Findings from a welfare-to-work demonstration project are described including enrollees who lose Medicaid but do not have employer-based health benefits.

INTRODUCTION

The problem of providing health care for the uninsured has recently regained national attention. A variety of approaches are being tried across the country including State High Risk Pools and other insurance pools, increasing individual policy options, and expansion of Medicaid and Medical Assistance eligibility. As a result there are new opportunities for involving Health Maintenance Organizations (HMOs) and other managed care systems in pro-

This chapter was originally published in *Journal of Health & Social Policy*, Vol. 1(1) 1989.

viding care to the uninsured. Findings of a demonstration project serving an uninsured workfare population are presented in later sections of this chapter.

Uninsured and uncompensated care have again taken top spots on the national, state, and local health policy agendas. However, these issues are not new on the American health care scene.[1] In the 1960s, the passage of Medicare and Medicaid brought sweeping changes by providing government sponsored insurance for the elderly, poor, and disabled.

Why then has the issue of the uninsured resurfaced so strongly? Of course, there is no single answer. Although Medicare and Medicaid provide benefits to a significant number of people, they simply do not cover all of the medical costs of the eligible elderly, disabled, or low-income population. Nor do they provide coverage for all of the uninsured. An insurance gap continues to exist.

Another important reason the issue of the uninsured has gained national attention is that competition and cost containment have radically changed the environment in which health care providers and insurers must operate. The shifting of uncompensated care costs by providers to private insurers and to Medicare and Medicaid has been greatly restricted. These two trends, demand for services, and the tightening of the reimbursement/financing system have elevated the problem of the uninsured to that of a major policy issue.

Who Are the Uninsured?

There is a general expectation in this country that families get health insurance coverage through their employers as a basic employment benefit. While the relative contributions to premiums, copayments, and deductibles vary, the trend, until recently, has been toward more comprehensive coverage paid in large part by the employer. While it is true that the unemployed and their dependents are likely to be uninsured, it is the employed and their dependents who comprise three-quarters of the uninsured in this country. National figures estimate 30-35 million Americans are without insurance.[2] Some argue that this estimate may understate the number of people who have inadequate or only partial coverage.[3] Nonetheless, it is clear that the lack of employer-based coverage leaves 16-17 million employees and their families without health insurance.[4] Solutions must address this group.

The Risky Working Poor

Sweeping changes are occurring across the country through welfare reform. New work incentive/workfare programs are being considered and implemented in many states and counties. The new workfare population is joining the ranks of the working poor who lose Medicaid coverage and yet do not have employer health benefits. Only very recently have welfare reform initiatives begun considering the impact on the health system and the potential failures due to poor health and the lack of insurance.

While the health care needs of this group may not be as demanding or expensive as the high risk population considered uninsurable, it is still a risky group. The low-income population generally has a lower health status. As former Medicaid recipients, workfare participants have a history of using more services and more expensive services than the general population. As former Medicaid recipients, they are also likely to have a history of inappropriate use of the health care system, of not having had a primary care physician, and of relying on episodic emergency room care. When enrolling a workfare group, insurers, including prepaid plans, can expect to face high utilization costs which may not come down for as much as two years.[5] Providers have also expressed concern about compliance and continuity of care problems.

Managed care has been used in Medicaid programs in order to overcome problems similar to those of the working poor. These include lack of access to primary care, use of costly emergency rooms, doctor shopping, excessive testing and prescriptions, and high inpatient hospital use.[6] Ed Neuschler, at the National Governor's Association, has conducted a review of Medicaid Managed Care programs. He found that while most of these initiatives have not been operational long enough, managed care is a promising approach to cost and access/quality issues. There are some savings and few significant access/quality complaints.[7]

POTENTIAL MANAGED CARE INVOLVEMENT

Federal, state, and local governments are actively considering what their role might be in managed care, and how to promote private sector responses. Some states and localities are already contracting directly with HMOs on behalf of specific uninsured groups. In the public sector, a number of approaches are being developed and implemented including: (1) direct payments to providers for uncompensated care; (2) direct subsidies to individuals to purchase services/coverage; (3) promoting expanded coverage through existing public and private insurance mechanisms; (4) direct offering of government organized groups for health insurance purposes, (5) government contracts with private entities for services, particularly for managed care systems. An increasing number of states are sponsoring High Risk Pools for people considered medically uninsurable under standard plans. Expansion of Medicaid eligibility and opportunities for individuals to buy into a Medicaid-based plan are also options being considered by states. States are gaining experience using managed care (particularly HMOs) for their Medicaid recipients.

On the private sector side, there is a need and a potential market for new health benefit packages specifically for small firms and for employed uninsured individuals. While these types of firms and individuals have not traditionally been considered desirable, carefully designed products could open new markets, particularly for HMOs. The need is there; the interest is there; and so is the risk.

Key Design Issues

There are many elements to consider within the design and administration of health benefit packages for the uninsured including: eligibility, financing/subsidies, the benefit package, cost controls, the use of managed care, quality of care, and administration. These are briefly discussed below and then later highlighted through a discussion of a welfare-to-work demonstration project in Maryland.

Eligibility

The term "uninsured" is used loosely in a number of different contexts. However, for the purposes of designing a health insurance package for the uninsured, a distinction should be made between medically high risk uninsurables, the employed uninsured, the employed underinsured, and the unemployed uninsured. These are very different groups with different medical needs and financial means. High risk uninsurables are generally those individuals considered medically uninsurable due to pre-existing medical conditions. They are usually ineligible for coverage through employer groups or as individuals. A number of states have implemented High Risk Pools for the medically uninsurable which allow these individuals to purchase health insurance coverage through the pool. HMOs should be aware that states are beginning to consider managed care and HMO contracts for the Risk Pools. The unemployed uninsured are likely to have serious financial constraints and present marketing problems for the plan. The employed uninsured and underinsured and their employers, on the other hand, may be interested in purchasing coverage if it is tailored to their needs.

Financing and Subsidies

Affordability is a key issue for all of these uninsured populations. Experience to date, with High Risk Pools, suggests that government subsidies are unavoidable if premiums are to be within reach of the eligible population.[8] One alternative that states are considering is to create larger pools which would include other uninsured groups as well as the high risk uninsured. This model is appealing because the risk could be spread across a larger and probably healthier group. Premiums for the high risk group would probably be lower. However, premiums for the other uninsured groups would probably be higher than if they were in a separate pool.

Because of the intense interest in uncompensated care and increasing awareness and sophistication on the part of employers, it is conceivable that public subsidies and/or new employer contributions might be available to cover part of the premium costs of a benefit package tailored to people who would otherwise be uninsured. The level and mix of these funding sources will vary considerably depending on the local situation and state level activities. Nonetheless, these possibilities should be investigated, if not directly negotiated.

Benefit Package

Comprehensive group-style benefits have become a norm in this country. However, given the costs of these plans, other benefits designs should be considered such as the "low end" benefit package recommended by Bovbjerg.[9] The range of benefits offered can usually be tailored to meet the needs of the group. For example, the plan could offer dental, vision care, and pharmacy coverage or it could exclude expensive mental health and addiction services. Decisions about benefit coverage can greatly affect price and the usefulness of the coverage to the beneficiaries.

Cost Control

Virtually every insurer builds in cost control mechanisms such as utilization review, pre-admission certification, and fee screens. These controls affect services provided to the patient and can foster appropriate use of services and keep premium increases to a minimum. HMOs are in an excellent position to use their existing cost control mechanisms to provide services to this population group. They provide immediate access to primary care physicians, but also promote case management and cost controls.

Managed Care Options

As was noted above, the use of managed care is closely tied to cost control mechanisms, and is critical to the success of benefit packages for the uninsured. A number of costly utilization patterns, such as inappropriate emergency room and inpatient care, can be reduced by promoting coordination, continuity of care, and prevention. At the same time enrollee access to primary care can be improved. There are a number of alternative approaches to managed care such as Primary Care Case Managers (based on fee for service plus a management fee), Health Insuring Organizations (HIOs) and Health Maintenance Organizations (HMOs).[10] HMOs, again, are in an advantageous position because of their experience and success with existing managed care approaches.

Quality Assurance

With the expected emphasis on cost controls, quality assurance mechanisms must also be in place. This can be part of a utilization review or peer review program and should include grievance mechanisms for both enrollees and providers. The plan purchaser should be confident that the cost control mechanisms do not result in poor quality care or inappropriate under service.

THE FAMILY INDEPENDENCE PROJECT (FIP) DEMONSTRATION

The remainder of this chapter will describe a county-based welfare-to-work program addressing health and health insurance problems of their clients. This is a joint public/private sector initiative which assures health benefit coverage for a target group of employed low-income workers and their families. The program, the Family Independence Project (FIP), assists teen parents and long-term Aid to Families with Dependent Children (AFDC) welfare recipients to secure employment and become self-sufficient.

The Health Component

The health component is a critical element of the overall project. The health component provides clients with private sector HMO benefit coverage as well as supplemental health promotion and health education through the Center for Prepaid Health Care Research. The Center for Prepaid Health Care Research is a private non-profit organization which is under contract with the county to provide the health component services.

The health benefits component of FIP is designed to address four of the most difficult problems for former welfare recipients:

1. the lack of adequate health benefit coverage;
2. dependence on publicly subsidized health care;
3. the lower health status associated with low-income people; and

4. the inappropriate use of health care services generally associated with Medicaid recipients.

The Model

The model used in this project has several important features: (1) its enrollment of a welfare-to-work population; (2) the use of a Non-Profit Group Administrator; (3) the use of multiple funding sources and subsidies; (4) the use of managed care; and (5) the provision of proactive health promotion and education services. These are discussed below.

Eligibility. For purposes of the demonstration project, eligibility is limited to participants in the Family Independence Project (FIP). This group probably typifies the working poor and also has many of the characteristics of the Medicaid population.

The Non-Profit Group Administrator. In this demonstration project, the Center for Prepaid Health Care Research acts as the group administrator for the FIP population, much as a personnel department provides this service to a business' employees. The Center is also responsible for providing appropriate health promotion and education services. These arrangements are unique among programs of this type.

Subsidies/Financing. One of the most innovative aspects of the program is the group administrator's ability to use multiple funding sources. Premium payments for this demonstration project come from a combination of county funds, employers, participants, and other sources. Currently, once a participant becomes ineligible for Medicaid, premium subsidies are provided for a limited time. In the future it is hoped that arrangements can be made to cover the costs for Medicaid-eligible participants through a capitated arrangement with the State Medicaid Office.

The flexibility to change the proportion of the premium payments paid by each source is the most attractive feature to those funding sources. The enrollees are expected to contribute to premium costs in proportion to their income. Employer contributions are negotiated. When participant and employer contributions do not cover the premium costs, county funding and corporate or philanthropic contributions are used by the Center.

Contracting with an HMO. The Center contracts with an existing

HMO, M.D.IPA (Medical Doctors Independent Practice Association), for a standard group policy. In order to negotiate such a contract for a risky group just off of Medicaid, the other program components were persuasive. The additional health promotion and health education activities are specifically being used to address problems of low health status and inappropriate use of the health care system.

Experience to Date

The Family Independence Project (FIP) began enrolling participants in April of 1986. Health promotion/health education activities began shortly after the first enrollments and continued intensively through the summer and fall of 1986. Preliminary data allows us to: (1) describe the basic demographic characteristics of the FIP participants; (2) determine self-reported health status and health care utilization; and (3) identify the most common lifestyle patterns affecting health status of the participants. The following information is current as of April 1988.

Demographic Characteristics

The average age of the participants is 29.2 and only 14 of the participants are currently teen parents. On average, participants completed eleven years of school.

Generally, the FIP participants are somewhat older and better educated than was expected based on the characteristics of the county's AFDC population. The racial composition of half black does generally reflect the county's AFDC population except that more Hispanic and Asian participants were expected. The preliminary data show that nearly two-thirds of the participants were teenagers at the birth of their first child.

Self-Reported Health Status and Health Care Utilization

Applicants to FIP are asked a series of questions by the case manager in order to obtain baseline information on perceived health status, health care utilization, and family planning. The following is based on 180 applicants, some of whom may have subsequently left the program, but the majority of whom became active participants. Where possible this data is compared to a 1986 national survey on access to health care conducted by the Robert Wood Johnson Foundation (RWJ).[11]

Health Status. Clients were asked to rank their health on a four-point scale. Twenty-eight percent (28%) ranked themselves as "Excellent"; 28% as "Very Good"; 35% as "Good"; and 8% as "Fair." RWJ reported 12% of the total population said "Fair" or "Poor." Nationally, 10.5% of the 17-64-year-olds ranked "Fair" or "Poor."

Medical Emergencies. Approximately 34% of the respondents' families experienced a medical emergency in the last year, and 90% went to a hospital emergency room. The most frequently sighted reason for using the emergency room was that it was nearby. The recent RWJ survey found nationally an average of 18% of families with an emergency visit in the past 12 months.

Primary Care. When asked if there was a time when you didn't get medical care when you needed it, 88% said no and 12% said yes. The most frequently sighted reasons for not obtaining care were lack of money and that the provider did not accept Medicaid. Similarly, the RWJ survey found 16% of the population not getting care for financial reasons. Eighteen percent of our respondents do not have a regular source of care. Nationally, 22.3% of 17-64-year-olds reported not having a regular source of care. When ill, 13% of our respondents reported using a hospital emergency room.

Respondents are more likely to have a regular source of care for their children (93%) than they are for themselves (78%). In fact, 76% said they take their child to a doctor's office or clinic when they are ill. About 5% reported they would use a hospital emergency room for their children when they are sick. Nationally, 9.9% of children, compared to 7% of FIP children do not have a regular source of care.

Chronic Illness and Disability. FIP participants are not expected to have many disabilities because they are relatively young. However, nearly thirty-one percent (31%) reported a chronic illness and six percent (6%) of them said that they had to make changes in their lives in the last year due to medical problems. This appears to be high compared to the RWJ survey. Although different questions were used by RWJ, the estimated nation's chronic illness rate was 19.4% for 17-64-year-olds and 7.8% for children under 17.

Family Planning. Respondents were asked if they wanted information on family planning. Eighty percent (80%) said no, 20% said yes. Of those who did not want information, only 68% were currently using birth control.

Lifestyle Characteristics

All participants were given a health risk assessment. The findings of the health risk assessment were then used for follow-up counseling. During the course of the counseling sessions, participants were asked to identify several activities that they would modify or add to their daily lives in order to reduce their risk of disease and disability. These personal goals ranged from using seat belts to eating whole wheat toast for breakfast to exercising three times a week. In the aggregate, the major and most common problems were stress management, nutrition, and exercise.

Opinion of Medical Care Received

Respondents were asked to rate the medical care they have received on a four-point scale (fine as is, needs improvement, not satisfactory, not sure). Their responses were based on several aspects of medical care including quality, willingness of the doctor to discuss and explain the problem and treatment, amount of time to get an appointment, office waiting time, respect and courtesy, and ease of getting emergency care. Overall, respondents ratings were positive: 82% found their health care "fine as is," 15% felt it "needs improvement" and 1% said it was "not satisfactory." RWJ found a satisfaction rate of 74.3%.

Previous Health Insurance Coverage

Sixty-nine percent (69%) of the 180 respondents had never had any medical coverage other then Medicaid. Those who had had other kinds of coverage in the past had benefits through an employer.

CONCLUSION

The problems of the uninsured are getting worse because of the competitive, cost-containment-oriented environment in which health care providers must now operate. Solutions must be diverse and innovative in order to deal with this complex issue. A variety of approaches, including managed care and HMO contracting, are being considered by governments and the private sector.

The demonstration project described here is a unique approach using public and private sources, and case management. This welfare-to-work group is similar to other uninsured groups in that they are young, less educated, and working in low-income less technical occupations. Guaranteed health benefit coverage improves access while acting as an incentive to get off of welfare.

Participants' self-perceived health status is equal to or higher than the general population. However, the high rates of chronic conditions and emergency room use while participants were on Medicaid, suggest the need for stronger relationships with a primary care physician as well as education and/or assistance in managing health problems. Managed care delivery systems offer excellent options for addressing these needs.

REFERENCE NOTES

1. Theodore R. Marmor, *Politics of Medicare* (Chicago: Aldine Publishing Co., 1970).

2. Gail R. Wilinsky, "Whose Care is Uncompensated and What are the Key Options," a paper presented at the National Health Council: Washington Briefing on Uncompensated Care, Washington, DC, October 10, 1985; Daniel C. Walden, Gail R. Wilinsky, and Judith A. Kasper, "Changes in Health Insurance Status: Full Year and Part Year Coverage," *National Health Care Expenditure Study* (Bethesda, MD: National Center for Health Services Research and Health Care Technology Assessment) Data Preview 21, DHS Publication No. (PHS-85-337); Margaret B. Sulvetta, and Katherine Swartz, *The Uninsured and Uncompensated Care: A Chart Book* (Washington, DC: George Washington University, National Health Policy Forum, June 1986); American Hospital Association, *Cost and Compassion: Recommendations for Avoiding a Crisis in Care for the Medically Indigent* (Chicago: American Hospital Association, 1986), pp. 113-114.

3. American Hospital Association, p. 103.

4. American Hospital Association, p. 104.

5. Karen Wintringham and Thomas W. Bice, "Effects of Turnover on Use of Services by Medicaid Beneficiaries in a Health Maintenance Organization," *The Group Health Journal*, Spring 1985, pp. 12-18.

6. Edward Neuschler, "Overview of Medicaid Managed Health Care Initiatives," prepared for the Forum on Prepaid Capitation Programs for Medicaid Recipients, Albuquerque, New Mexico, October 28, 1985 (Washington, DC: The National Governors Association, 1985), p. 1.

7. Neuschler, p. 19.

8. Randall R. Bovbjerg and Christopher F. Koller, "State Health Insurance Pools: Current Performance, Future Prospects," *Inquiry*, 23(2): 111-121, 1986.

9. Randall R. Bovbjerg, "Insuring the Uninsured Through Private Action: Ideas and Initiatives," *Inquiry*, 23(4) 412-413, 1986.

10. For a review of the range of managed care alternatives see Edward Neuschler, "Overview of Medicaid Managed Health Care Initiatives," prepared for the Forum on Prepaid Capitation Programs for Medicaid Recipients, Albuquerque, New Mexico, October 28, 1985 (Washington, DC: The National Governors Association, 1985).

11. Robert Wood Johnson Foundation, "Access to Health Care in the United States: Results of a 1986 Survey," Special Report Number Two/1987 (Princeton, New Jersey: Robert Wood Johnson Foundation).

PLANNING ISSUES

Services to populations at risk are limited in every community, and no community can fully respond to all of the perceived needs and demands people may make. Assessments must be made in regard to how much responsibility communities can take in when resources are limited and distribution is frequently politically motivated. We tend to struggle with marketplace-driven factors, that is the consumer in the best position to determine how much money he should spend on health care. All things equal, many consumers are forced to decide whether they should purchase health care or pay the rent. Planning also takes into consideration location access, and relative need of service. There are a number of populations that require special consideration in the planning process. Homeless women and ambulatory patients with human immunodeficiency syndrome infections will be examined in this section. In addition, computerized need projection and psychological factors as predictors will also be examined.

Chapter 5

Designing Services for Homeless Women

Jan L. Hagen

SUMMARY. The complexity of homelessness suggests that the development of policy and service strategies requires careful analysis of the unique features of identifiable groups within the homeless population. To begin this process, the characteristics and needs of homeless women are specified and their routes to homelessness delineated. Responses to homeless women, with the exception of battered women, have focused primarily on the provision of emergency services. Future policy and services must focus on the adequacy and accessibility of these emergency services as well as the need for transitional and long-term housing and social services. The multidimensional nature of homelessness and the heterogeneity of homeless women require a wide range of alternatives that can e tailored to each woman's unique need for service.

Emerging as a significant social problem in the early 1980s (Stern, 1984), homelessness has become a pressing concern for social service providers, policy analysts, politicians, and the general public. Paralleling this concern has been an increase in research on the characteristics and needs of homeless people. As the traditional image of the homeless person as an older, white male alcoholic living on skid row gave way to an image of "bag ladies" and "grate men," much of this research focused on homeless people who are chronically mentally ill. Only recently has the increasing diversity of the homeless population been widely recognized, leading numerous sources to conclude that the hallmark of today's homeless

This chapter was originally published in *Journal of Health & Social Policy*, Vol. 1(3) 1990.

population is its heterogeneity (Hagen, 1987b; Hopper, 1984; Stoner, 1984).

Beginning in the 1970s, the homeless population began to include not only the older, white male alcoholic but also women of all ages as well as younger men; minorities were overrepresented (Hopper & Hamberg, 1984). This trend toward a more diverse homeless population has continued. Nationwide, families now comprise an estimated 20 percent of the homeless population, and this trend toward more homeless families is expected to continue (Basler, 1986).

The complexity of homelessness requires that subpopulations of homeless persons be isolated in order to develop policy and service strategies responsive to the multiple needs and diverse characteristics of those who are homeless (Roth & Bean, 1986). To begin this process, this article focuses on homeless women, one subgroup identified as being acutely at risk and highly vulnerable (Farr, 1986; Roth, Toomey, & First, n.d.; Stoner, 1983). The characteristics and needs of homeless women are specified, routes to homelessness delineated, current responses examined, and future policy and service directions considered.

TODAY'S HOMELESS WOMEN

Although research on homelessness is increasing rapidly, relatively little of it has been focused exclusively or primarily on homeless women. (Exceptions include the works of Bassuk, Rubin, & Lauriat, 1986; Corrigan & Anderson, 1984; Crystal, 1984; Hagen, 1987a; Stark, 1986; and Strasser, 1978.) Even an estimated percentage of homeless people who are women is difficult to obtain. Some studies indicate that women comprise 15 to 20 percent of the homeless population while others have documented a much higher percentage (Hagen, 1987b; Rossi et al., 1987; Roth et al., 1985; Slavinsky & Cousins, 1982). These differences, of course, may be explained by sampling procedures. When families as well as women residing in battered women shelters are included, the data indicate that women now comprise about one-half of the homeless population.

In recent years, the bulk of the research on homelessness has been primarily cross-sectional, descriptive-correlational studies using a variety of survey methods. To make this research accessible to analysis, a typology of homeless people based on the work of Breakey and Fischer (1986) will be used to highlight findings relevant to homeless women. These three groups are the chronically mentally ill, chronic alcoholics, and the situationally homeless. The situationally homeless "are those whose homelessness has resulted from a change in circumstances, such as unemployment, spousal abuse, eviction, or urban redevelopment" (Breakey, 1987, p. 42). This group is sometimes referred to as the "new homeless." Although useful for analysis, these categories must be used with some caution. Stoner (1984) makes the astute observation that by distinguishing between the "new homeless" and the "chronic homeless," public policy and newly developed services for the homeless may come to reflect the tradition of the Elizabethan Poor Laws in their categorization of the "worthy" and "unworthy" poor.

Chronically Mentally Ill

Much of the attention directed toward homelessness has focused on homeless people who are chronically mentally ill. A highly visible group, the mentally ill are generally regarded as constituting between 25 and 50 percent of homeless adults (Arce & Vergare, 1984). Although estimates vary widely (see, for example, Snow et al., 1986; Lipton, Sabatini, & Katz, 1983), Vergare and Arce (1986) have suggested that the precise percentage of homeless people who are chronically mentally ill is less important than the recognition that many homeless adults suffer from serious psychiatric disorders.

Although little attention has been given to differences between homeless men and women who are chronically mentally ill, gender differences have been noted in several studies. In two separate studies conducted in New York City shelters (Crystal & Goldstein, 1984a; 1984b), women were twice as likely as men to have psychiatric histories or indications of mental illness (47 percent vs. 22 percent). In a special study of homeless women in New York City shelters, Crystal (1984) found over half (53.3 percent) of the women had histories of previous psychiatric hospitalizations, were current psychiatric outpatients, or were assessed as having psychiatric problems. Bassuk, Rubin, and Lauriat (1984) also have noted gender differences among guests in a Boston shelter.

In contrast, however, a large-scale study in Ohio found homeless men and women to have similar levels of psychiatric impairment based on scores from the Psychiatric Status Schedule (Roth, Toomey, & First, n.d.). Additionally, findings from an Albany, New York study indicated no gender differences for homeless mentally ill persons as assessed by the agency's professional staff (Hagen, 1987a). Finally, a Massachusetts study of sheltered homeless families concluded that, although "one-fourth of the mothers were assigned DSM-III Axis-I diagnoses indicating the presence of major psychiatric clinical syndromes" (including 9 percent with substance abuse diagnoses), "psychoses were not overrepresented among homeless mothers" (Bassuk, Robin, & Lauriat, 1986, pp. 1098, 1100).

Regarded as characteristic of homeless people generally, disaffiliation from family, friends, and social roles is even more noticeable among the mentally ill (Bassuk, Robin, & Lauriat, 1984). For women with children, however, disaffiliation may be experienced somewhat differently. Crystal (1984, pp. 5-6) notes that although separated from their children, many homeless women "maintain some kind of ongoing parental relationship . . . and the majority hoped . . . to resume caretaking for them." He concluded that many of the women seemed removed from the disaffiliated image and that "children represent a still-vital link of kinship which belies the 'disaffiliation' image." Crystal's conclusion has been supported further in a study by Hagen and Ivanoff (1988) in which one-half of the homeless women identified close personal relationships.

Additional research on mental disorders among homeless people raises two interrelated points. First, although Bassuk and her colleagues (1986, p. 1100) found 71 percent of the homeless mothers in a family shelter study to have personality disorders, they point out that:

> . . . personality disorder is a diagnosis of social dysfunction and does not take into account the influence of environmental factors extrinsic to the organization of the personality, such as poverty, racism, and gender-bias. Criteria for these disorders

are no more than descriptions of behavioral disturbances that are long-term and predate the homeless episode. The resultant diagnostic labeling may exaggerate the degree of psychopathology within this subgroup of homeless women. Thus, the labels should primarily be used to indicate severe functional impairment and the need for help rather than implying strict causality.

Second, some research suggests that mental disorders among homeless people may be a consequence of homelessness itself, accompanied as it is by such associated factors as extreme poverty, job loss, limited social supports, harsh environmental conditions, assault, and sexual abuse (Robertson, 1986). The importance of relationships to most women and the vulnerability of homeless women to sexual exploitation and rape suggest an increased risk for psychological distress and impairment among homeless women.

Chronic Alcoholics

Although this subgroup of homeless people was studied extensively in the past, relatively few studies in recent years have focused exclusively on homeless chronic alcoholics. And, as has been the tradition in alcohol-related research, women alcoholics have received even less attention.

Stark's (1987, p. 11) comprehensive review of alcoholism studies from 1980 through 1986 revealed an alcohol abuse rate averaging 30 to 33 percent among the homeless population and "this rate has remained stable, not only through time but also geographically and situationally. . . ." Thus, alcohol abuse remains a key factor contributing to homelessness.

Several studies have noted gender differences in rates of alcohol abuse. For example, an Ohio study found 24 percent of the men had chronic alcohol problems compared to 7 percent of the women (Roth, Toomey, & First, n.d.). An Albany, New York study of 227 homeless individuals or families requesting services from a centralized intake agency for the homeless reported alcohol abuse for 16 percent of the men compared to 9 percent of the women (Hagen, 1987a).

Few studies report other types of substance abuse. However, the

Albany intake study (Hagen, 1987a) found drug abuse among 3.6 percent of the men compared to 1 percent of the women and the New York City shelter study (Crystal & Goldstein, 1984b) noted regular hard drug usage for 4.7 percent of the men and 2 percent of the women. Several studies on homeless women have also noted rates of substance abuse. In the Massachusetts study of sheltered families, 8 percent of the mothers had alcohol problems and 9 percent had drug problems (Bassuk, Rubin, & Lauriat, 1986). Although alcohol and drug abuse are more likely to be problems experienced by homeless men, substance abuse figures significantly as a contributing factor in the homelessness of women.

Situationally Homeless

Relatively little research has been conducted on today's situationally homeless. For this group, the problem of homelessness has been regarded as primarily financial. Their problems "stem from failure to cope with difficult circumstances, not so much from major disabilities like mental illness or alcoholism" (Breakey & Fischer, 1985, p. 20). While there are a myriad of reasons for homelessness among this group, several are key: unemployment, poverty, scarcity of affordable housing, and family disruption, including domestic violence. Given the types of difficulties leading to homelessness for this group, it can be hypothesized that women alone as well as those with children are a disproportionate component of this category.

Again, widely varying estimates of the situationally homeless emerge, ranging from 20 percent to 70 percent (Crystal, 1984; Hagen, 1985). In large part, this variation is explained by sampling procedures. Families are often housed outside homeless shelters and, thus, would be excluded in these surveys. Additionally, if those with mental illness, including alcoholism, are less likely to remain tied to the formal delivery system, the situationally homeless are more likely to appear in surveys of social service agencies.

While the lack of affordable, safe housing has been well documented, relatively little attention has been given to the relationship between poverty and homelessness. Poverty alone places people at risk for homelessness and particularly at risk for poverty are female-headed households who are heavily dependent on inadequate public assistance benefits. Over the last decade, the relative value of incomes generally has declined and public assistance benefits particularly have failed to keep pace with inflation. Public assistance recipients commonly make rent payments in excess of their allotted shelter allowances.

The differential participation and earnings of women in the labor force are well documented. By contributing to low income and poverty for women, unemployment and underemployment increase the risk for homelessness and, once homeless, make securing adequate housing difficult.

Family disruption also makes women and their children vulnerable to homelessness, particularly those who have limited financial resources. Family violence, especially wife battering, may result in the establishment of single-parent families needing independent housing. The potential enormity of this problem is reflected in the estimate that about 1.8 million wives are abused by their husbands each year (Straus & Gelles, 1986).

Although research on the situationally homeless is only beginning, several studies have noted gender differences. Hagen (1987a) reports that women are more likely to experience homelessness as a result of domestic violence and eviction than men. In their study of homeless women, Hagen and Ivanoff (1988) identified a total of 66 percent as situationally homeless, primarily due to family difficulties (including 22 percent who were victims of domestic violence), and economic factors such as unemployment. Roth and her colleagues (n.d., p. 7) also noted economic factors and family problems as central reasons for homelessness among women:

> Over 40 percent cited economic factors such as unemployment, problems paying rent, eviction or benefits being terminated as the primary reason for their loss of a permanent home. However, for almost an equal percentage of women, family conflict or dissolution resulted in their being homeless.
>
> In contrast, only 18 percent of men attributed their homelessness to family difficulties.

In summary, although knowledge regarding homeless women is limited, there are indications that homeless women are somewhat more likely than homeless men to be mentally ill and to have previously experienced psychiatric hospitalization. Homeless women are less likely than homeless men to experience difficulties with alcohol and drug abuse and to be disaffiliated from family, friends, and social roles. The much discussed and documented "feminization of poverty" and the more recent attention to the "pauperization of children" indicate that women and their children are at particularly high risk for homelessness due to poverty and, once homeless, locating affordable housing becomes exceedingly difficult. Family dissolution and family violence also place women at increased risk for homelessness.

DEVELOPING A SERVICE CONTINUUM

The major strategy for responding to homeless people has been the provision of emergency shelter and food by voluntary agencies. Food pantries, soup kitchens, drop-in centers, and shelters are sponsored by such organizations as churches, the Red Cross, and Travelers Aid as well as agencies that have traditionally provided missions such as the Salvation Army. In the public sector, local governments increasingly are responding to the needs of homeless people by providing shelters. However, the intensely politicized nature of homelessness has resulted in no coherent response at the local level (Ropers, 1985).

Further, although examples exist of innovative efforts by the voluntary sector and state governments which demonstrate a broadening of concern from the provision of emergency shelter to more long-term solutions, they are isolated instances and do not reflect a comprehensive strategy for addressing homelessness. The service system is characterized not only by insufficient, and in many instances inadequate, shelter facilities but also by tremendous fragmentation of services. In addition to the lack of coordination, such issues as accessibility, acceptability, adequacy, and accountability have yet to be addressed.

Comprehensive approaches to public policy for homelessness propose a three-tiered continuum of services moving from the emergency responses of shelter, food, and financial assistance to transitional services including housing assistance, employment assistance, and health, mental health, and social services. The final tier is envisioned as stabilization: permanent housing, either independent or in supportive environments with supplemental services provided as required (Kaufman, 1984). One strength of this model is the rational sequencing of needed services that can accommodate the diverse groups of homeless individuals and families. At the transition and stabilization tiers particularly, service responses can be tailored to the needs of various groups of homeless people, from alcoholics to the mentally ill to victims of domestic violence. The individualization of interventions at these two tiers appears crucial if a recurrence of homelessness is to be avoided. However, effective interventions at these levels requires both the coordination of the existing services as well as the development of such missing components as housing alternatives, training and employment services, health services, and mental health services.

By highlighting available services as well as deficiencies, a three-tiered continuum of services begins to frame the policy agenda at the local, state, and national levels. Using this continuum, it becomes readily apparent, for example, that transitional and supportive housing for alcoholics, the elderly, and victims of domestic violence are not readily available in most communities. Additionally, a three-tiered continuum of services facilitates the identification of minimally acceptable standards at each tier. (See Stoner, 1983, for an illustration.) These in turn serve to guide policy and program developments, particularly at the local level where services are actually delivered.

In her three-tiered continuum of services, Kaufman (1984, p. 22) proposes two additional and essential components: prevention and case management as the critical link between tiers, as "the glue which holds the continuum together." A focus on prevention serves to highlight risk factors for homelessness such as inadequate levels of financial assistance, lack of low income housing, structural unemployment, and inadequate community-based services for the chronically mentally ill. Primary prevention would focus on broadly based policy changes mainly at the state and federal levels. To the extent that individuals and families encountering these risks can be identified, such actions as supplemental rent payments and outreach can be taken to prevent homelessness.

Envisioning the case manager as the link between the three tiers, Kaufman (1984, p. 23) defines the case manager as someone who can "mobilize the resources necessary to assist a person out of the crisis and on the road to stabilization" as well as a provider of mental health services. To fulfill these functions, the case manager must have considerable autonomy as well as the freedom to function outside a formal agency setting. It can be anticipated that caseloads will need to be limited given the multiple needs of homeless individuals and families and that work with many clients will be on a long-term basis.

Proch and Taber (1987, p. 8), as well as others, consider the first tier of emergency shelter as the primary need of homeless people. The whys of homelessness are irrevelant to the need for shelter and "until people have shelter, attempts to address the many factors that may contribute to the need for shelter are premature." Proch and Taber's conservative estimate for assuring minimal shelter is $1.5 billion (excluding capital expenditures for developing shelter facilities). Revenues of this magnitude must be provided by state and federal governments and, because homelessness is not a temporary problem, funding should be provided on an ongoing basis rather than through emergency appropriations.

Because of the prevailing pattern of far fewer shelter facilities for homeless women than men, priority should be given to developing shelters accessible and acceptable to homeless women, including respectful, simple admission procedures and provisions for privacy and autonomy (Koegel, 1986). The growth of homeless families, most of whom are mother-only families, requires extensive development of emergency family shelters. Obtaining emergency shelter should in no instance require separating family members.

In addition to shelter, the emergency response to homeless women must also include two additional components. First, outreach services are needed for those who, because of impaired mental capacity, may not seek shelter on their own (Roth, Toomey, & First, n.d.). The reported higher rates of mental disorders among homeless women indicate they may have a greater need for outreach services than homeless men. Second, crisis services are required for those who are situationally homeless due to family conflict or dissolution (including family violence), eviction, and recent unemployment. Hagen (1987a) has documented the increased risk for homelessness because of eviction for women and both Hagen

(1987a) and Roth, Toomey, and First (n.d.), have noted family conflict or dissolution as a central reason for homelessness among women. In addition to crisis counseling, the major service needs may be assistance in locating affordable housing and accessing public assistance benefits.

For some women, the provision of these emergency services may be sufficient. For situationally homeless women, homelessness has the *potential* of being a short-term phenomenon. Results from the Ohio study suggest that one-third to one-half of all homeless women can fairly quickly return to independent living (Roth, Toomey, & First, n.d.). Given adequate financial resources and available, affordable housing, some situationally homeless women do not require supplemental services or assistance in the long term to live independently.

Transitional services are needed by a wide range of homeless people–those with drug and alcohol difficulties, those requiring job retraining and job preparation, those without independent living skills, and those needing protective services such as domestic violence victims, the elderly, and the mentally ill. The Ohio study identified about one-third of the homeless women "as substantially impaired but restorable with a longer term of care delivered in a fairly vigorous program effort" (Roth, Toomey, & First, n.d., p. 16). The projected length of service ranges from six to eighteen months. In addition to rehabilitative and psychotherapeutic services, this group requires extensive social care services including access services such as information, referral, and advocacy as well as case management to coordinate the package of required services and to provide supportive counseling.

For homeless women, several areas of transitional services are noteworthy. First is the need to develop and target alcohol and drug treatment programs to homeless women. Women have been consistently underrepresented in publicly funded alcohol and drug treatment programs ("Study Finds," 1987). In providing these services to homeless women, two issues are central: (1) to provide not only detoxification and treatment, but also transitional housing in alcohol free environments with such supportive services as ongoing counseling, job training, and adequate financial resources; and (2) to develop treatment programs that acknowledge and support many alcoholic women's roles as mothers. Alcohol and drug treatment for alcoholic women need not be contingent on separating mothers from their children. An additional issue that will need to be addressed is the development of treatment facilities equipped to respond to dual addiction, a problem apparently more likely to be presented by women.

Second, some victims of domestic violence may need more than emergency services if they wish to leave an abusive relationship. Safe, transitional housing providing a protective environment will be required and, for those who have never worked or functioned as independent heads of households, additional supportive services will be required. Particularly important is financial independence either through employment or public assistance.

Third, transitional services will need to include a strong mental health component. The reported high levels of mental health symptoms among homeless people and the consistent finding that few receive mental health treatment suggest that mental health services must be more readily accessible not only to the homeless chronically mentally ill but also to those among the homeless with crisis and acute mental health needs.

The final tier of stabilization is permanent housing, either independent or supportive environments. The key here, of course, is to have available and affordable housing options for the diverse groups of homeless people. The development nationwide of low and moderate income housing is vital if the extent of homelessness is to be reduced. Of equal importance, however, is the recognition that some homeless people–those who are permanently outside the labor force, those with physical disabilities, those with chronic and severe mental disorders, and those with serious and long-term substance abuse histories–will always require supportive services, particularly case management, either within their housing facility or closely attached. Estimates indicate that up to one-third of the homeless individuals may require this type of long-term care (Redburn & Buss, 1986) and most of these will have chronic mental disorders. As Bachrach (1985, p. 1065) has noted, "severe psychopathology is more widespread and more intense among homeless women than homeless men." Further, Bassuk (1984, p. 45) notes:

... many chronically disturbed people simply cannot be rehabilitated, and the goal in these cases would be to provide the patient with comfortable and friendly asylum.

CONCLUSION

Homeless women and their children are a tremendous drain on public and private resources, including informal support networks. This pattern is likely to continue without coherent policies at the state and federal levels for major and multiple interventions that extend beyond the provision of emergency shelter and food. Combining and coordinating public and private efforts, interventions must address not only the much discussed mental health services needed by this population, but also the need for transitional living environments with supportive services for diverse groups of homeless women and their children—alcoholics and drug abusers, victims of domestic violence, young women and mothers without independent living skills, and the chronically mentally ill.

Some homeless women will be able to become independent given affordable and safe housing, available job opportunities at adequate wages, and adequate child support from noncustodial fathers. Others will require intensive, long-term supportive services as they move to increasing levels of independence. Additionally, we must recognize and address the needs of those who will require some degree of supportive services in the community throughout their lives. No single strategy for responding to homelessness is adequate for addressing the diverse and multiple needs of homeless women and their children. The multidimensional nature of homelessness and the heterogeneity of homeless women require a wide range of alternatives which can be tailored to each woman's unique needs for service.

REFERENCES

Arce, A.A. & Vergare, M.I. (1984). Identifying and characterizing the mentally ill among the homeless. In *The Homeless Mentally Ill* edited by H.R. Lamb. (pp. 75-89). Washington, DC: American Psychological Association.

Bachrach, L.I. (1985). Chronic mentally ill women: Emergence and legitimation of program issues. *Hospital and Community Psychiatry, 36,* 1063-1069.

Basler, B. (1986, January 12). Homeless families to double. *The New York Times,* p. 20.

Bassuk, E.L. (1984). The homelessness problem. *Scientific American, 251,* 40-45.

Bassuk, E.L., Rubin, L. & Lauriat, A. (1984). Is homelessness a mental health problem? *American Journal of Psychiatry, 141,* 1545-1550.

Bassuk, E.L., Rubin, L. & Lauriat, A. (1986). Characteristics of sheltered homeless families. *American Journal of Public Health, 76,* 1097-1101.

Breakey, W.R. (1987). Treating the homeless. *Alcohol Health and Research World, 11,* 42-46, 90.

Breakey, W.R. & Fischer, P.I. (1985, June). Down and out in the land of plenty. *Johns Hopkins Magazine,* 16-24.

Corrigan, E.M. & Anderson, S.C. (1984). Homeless alcoholic women on skid row. *American Journal of Drug and Alcohol Abuse, 10,* 535-549.

Crystal, S. (1984). Homeless men and homeless women: The gender gap. *Urban and Social Change Review, 17,* 2-6.

Crystal, S. & Goldstein, M. (1984a). *Correlates of Shelter Utilization: One day Study.* New York City Human Resources Administration.

Crystal, S. & Goldstein, M. (1984b). *The Homeless in New York City Shelters.* New York City Human Resources Administration.

Farr, R.K. (1986). A mental health treatment program for the homeless mentally ill in the Los Angeles skid row area. In *Treating the Homeless: Urban Psychiatry's Challenge,* edited by B.E. Jones (pp. 66-92). Washington, DC: American Psychiatric Press.

Fischer, P.I. & Breakey, W.R. (1986). Homelessness and mental health: An overview. *International Journal of Mental Health, 14,* 6-41.

Hagen, J.L. (1985). *Homelessness in the Capital District.* A report prepared for the Capital District Travelers Aid Society.

Hagen, I.L. (1987a). Gender and homelessness. *Social Work 32,* 312-316.

Hagen, J.L. (1987b). The heterogeneity of homelessness. *Social Casework, 68,* 451-457.

Hagen, J.L. & Ivanoff, A. (1988). Homeless women: A high-risk population. *Affilia: Journal of Women and Social Work, 3,* 19-33.

Hopper, K. (1984). Whose lives are these anyway? *Urban and Social Change Review, 17,* 12-13.

Hopper, K. & Hamberg, J. (1984). *The Making of America's Homeless: From Skid Row to New Poor, 1945-1984.* New York: New York Community Service Society.

Kaufman, N.K. (1984). Homelessness: A comprehensive policy approach. *Urban and Social Change Review, 17,* 21-26.

Koegel, P. (1986). *Ethnographic Perspectives on Homeless and Homeless Mentally Ill Women.* Proceedings of a two-day workshop sponsored by the Division of Education and Service Systems Liaison, National Institute of Mental Health.

Lipton, F.R., Sabatini, A., & Katz, S.E. (1983). Down and out in the city: The homeless mentally ill. *Hospital and Community Psychiatry, 34*, 817-821.

Proch, K. & Taber, M.A. (1987). Helping the Homeless. *Public Welfare, 45*, 5-9.

Redburn, F. S. & Buss, T.F. (1986). *Responding to America's Homeless: Public Policy Alternatives*. New York: Praeger.

Robertson, M.I. (1986). Mental disorders among homeless persons in the United States: An overview of recent empirical literature. *Administration in Mental Health, 14*, 14-27.

Ropers, R.H. (1985). The rise of the new urban homeless. *Public Affairs Report, 26*, 1-14.

Rossi, P.H., Wright, I.D., Fisher, G.A. & Willis, G. (1987). The urban homeless: Estimating composition and size. *Science, 235*, 1336-1341.

Roth, D. & Bean, G.I. (1986). New perspectives on homelessness: Findings from a statewide epidemiological study. *Hospital and Community Psychiatry, 37*, 712-719.

Roth, D., Toomey, B.G. & First, R.I. (no date). *Homeless Women: Characteristics and Service Needs of One of Society's Most Vulnerable Populations*. Columbus, Ohio: Department of Mental Health.

Roth, D., Bean, I., Lust, N. & Saveanu, T. (1985) *Homelessness in Ohio: A Study of People in Need*. Ohio Department of Mental Health.

Slavinsky, A.T. & Cousins, A. (1982). Homeless women. *Nursing Outlook, 30*, 358-362.

Snow, D.A., Baker, S.G., Anderson, L. & Martin, M. (1986). The myth of pervasive mental illness among the homeless. *Social Problems, 33*, 407-423.

Stark, L.R. (1986). Strangers in a strange land. *International Journal of Mental Health, 14*, 95-111.

Stark, L.R. (1987) A century of alcohol and homelessness: Demographics and stereotypes. *Alcohol Health and Research World, 11*, 8-13.

Stern, M.I. (1984). The emergence of the homeless as a public problem. *Social Service Review, 58*, 291-301.

Stoner, M.R. (1983). The plight of homeless women. *Social Service Review, 57*, 565-581.

Stoner, M.R. (1984). An analysis of public and private sector provisions for homeless people. *Urban and Social Change Review, 17*, 308.

Strasser, I.A. (1978). Urban transient women. *American Journal of Nursing, 78*, 2076-2079.

Straus, M.A. & Gelles, R.I. (1986). Societal change and change in family violence from 1975 to 1985 as revealed by two national surveys. *Journal of Marriage and the Family, 48*, 465-479.

Study finds women underrepresented in drug alcohol treatment programs. (1987). *American Journal of Public Health, 77*, 1357.

Vegare, M.I. & Arce, A.A. (1986). Homeless adult individuals and their shelter network. In *The Mental Health Needs of Homeless Persons*, edited by E.L. Bassuk. (pp. 15:26). San Francisco: Jossey-Bass.

Chapter 6

Mental Health Services Among Ambulatory Patients with Human Immunodeficiency Syndrome Infections

Kathleen Ell
David Larson
Wilbur Finch
Fred Sattler
Robert Nishimoto

SUMMARY. A retrospective study of 463 medical and social service records of patients with AIDS, ARC, and minimally symptomatic individuals was conducted to examine mental health services delivered by primary medical care providers. A substantial minority of patients in all three groups had a psychiatric diagnosis and were prescribed psychotropic medications. Recognition of psychiatric complications varied by ethnicity and socioeconomic status.

MENTAL HEALTH SERVICE USE AMONG AMBULATORY PATIENTS WITH HIV INFECTIONS

Between 1 and 2 million asymptomatic persons in the United States are believed to be infected with the Human Immunodefi-

The study was supported by contract No. 86 MO 198-319-01D from the National Institute of Mental Health.

This chapter was originally published in *Journal of Health & Social Policy*, Vol. 1(1) 1989.

ciency Virus (HIV). Up to 20-30% of these persons will eventually develop an AIDS (Acquired Immunodeficiency Syndrome)-Related Condition (ARC), and of those, approximately 15-20% will develop AIDS (Update, 1985; Jaffe et al., 1985). These projections may be conservative (Institute of Medicine, 1986; Chase, 1987). Currently, almost 50,000 Americans have been afflicted and more than one-half of these patients have died.

Despite the host of serious psychosocial problems already identified among patients with HIV, including frequently deteriorating functional status, lifestyle changes, neurologic impairment, the stress associated with having a fatal illness and mental disorders (Christ & Wiener, 1985; Baumgartner, 1985; Detmer, 1986-87; Holland & Tross, 1985), little is known about the mental health service utilization of these patients. For example, the majority of psychiatric studies have involved relatively small numbers of hospitalized patients with AIDS often selected by referral for psychiatric consultation of care (Nurnberg et al., 1984; Nichols, 1983; Perry & Jacobsen, 1986; Dilley et al., 1985; Perry & Markowitz, 1986; Wolcott et al., 1985; Faulstich, 1987).

Furthermore, there is a paucity of data comparing the mental health needs of ambulatory patients with AIDS versus ARC; although the latter group are frequently psychologically distressed due to the uncertainty as to whether they will develop AIDS (Holland & Tross, 1985). Finally, the extent to which observed psychiatric problems are associated with other potential predictors such as patients' sexual preference, social isolation, organic nervous system (CNS) disorders, HIV diagnostic categories, ethnicity and socioeconomic status (SES) has not been systematically examined.

It is especially disturbing that the majority of psychiatric studies have involved primarily Anglo middle- and upper-class patients since ethnic minority patients comprise approximately 40% of all patients with AIDS (Mays & Cochran, 1987). Moreover, among military applicants, ethnic minorities have higher rates of seropositivity for HIV than Anglos (Burke et al., 1987).

The striking gap in knowledge about mental health service utilization (Wolcott et al., 1986) among patients with HIV infections takes on even greater importance as the number of patients continues to escalate. Given the rapid increase in patients entering the health care system, it is likely that only a minority of patients will receive a formal psychiatric evaluation. It is far more likely that mental health services will be provided by primary care physicians and social workers (Belmont, Mantell, & Spivak, 1985; Hankin & Oktay, 1979; Goldberg & Huxley, 1980). When psychiatric complications are diagnosed by primary medical care providers, however, it is possible that data reflect missed diagnoses. For example, primary care physicians recognize only a minor portion of mental disorders (usually less than 20%) detected by formal psychiatric evaluation (Hankin & Oktay, 1979; Goldberg & Huxley, 1980). Missed diagnosis might also occur because organic brain symptomatology, including AIDS dementia and opportunistic infections and tumors of the CNS, may be similar to manifestations of psychiatric illness (Detmer, 1986-87). Moreover, as in the case of other serious illnesses, differentiating depression and anxiety disorder from normal reactions to life threatening events may further confound recognition of psychiatric problems (Petty & Noyes, 1981).

To investigate the provision of mental health services by primary care physicians and social workers, a retrospective study was conducted of 463 medical and social service records of patients with AIDS or ARC and minimally symptomatic individuals currently receiving care at the Interdisciplinary AIDS Clinic at Los Angeles County-University of Southern California-Medical Center (LAC-USC). Specific objectives of the study were: (1) to compare medical care physician recognition of psychiatric problems among patients with AIDS, ARC, or minimal symptomatology, and (2) to examine whether there were differences in either psychiatric problem recognition, psychotropic medication prescription or social service use by diagnostic group, ethnicity and socioeconomic status (SES).

STUDY METHODS

Sample Selection

The LAC-USC Interdisciplinary AIDS Service Clinic opened in March 1985. This Clinic provides comprehensive health care for patients with minimally symptomatic HIV infections as well as those with minor opportunistic infections (e.g., oral thrush, onychomycosis, self-limited cutaneous herpes), ARC, and AIDS. This service is accomplished by both primary care services and specialty clinics. Depending on their needs, patients are referred to specialty clinics which are attended by consultants with expertise in infectious disease, pulmonary, hematology-oncology, neurology, ophthalmology, otorhinolaryngology, rectal surgery, and gastrointestinal problems. The Clinic staff coordinates all aspects of outpatient and inpatient management. Patients also participate in research protocols since LAC-USC Medical Center is one of the AIDS Treatment and Evaluation Units (ATEU) and a member of the California cooperative Treatment Group (CCTG) for AIDS research. All outpatient medical records of 463 patients attending the General AIDS Clinic during the period of November 1986 to February 1987 were reviewed. The sample, therefore, represents all patients who were actively attending the clinic during the study period.

Data Collection Instruments and Procedures

An instrument developed for a previous chart review of hospitalized patients with AIDS (Belmont, Mantell, & Spivak, 1985) was modified for use in abstracting diagnostic and treatment data from clinic medical records. Sociodemographic data was obtained from a self-administered questionnaire that all clinic patients are required to complete at the time of initial clinic registration. Data collected from this clinic record included demographic and social characteristics, history of sexually transmitted disease, number of sexual partners since 1978, and drug use. In addition, psychological status as assessed by primary medical care physicians and psychotropic medications prescribed for clinic patients by their primary care physicians were abstracted from the clinic record.

Data collection was designed to allow for multiple diagnoses and treatments (up to five per clinic visit) and multiple clinic visits (up to 12 separate visits). Psychiatric diagnoses included anxiety, depression, and an "all other psychiatric problem" category. Psychotropic medications included anti-anxiety agents, anti-depressants, anti-psychotics, and sedative-hypnotics. Social work data were extracted from the Statistical Reporting Form utilized by clinic social workers. Data were categorized on this form as: (1) a problem in adjustment to illness, (2) an environmental problem, and (3) whether the patient or family was seen and (4) whether a community agency was contacted. Social workers followed clinic patients in the hospital and their records do not distinguish in-hospital visits from clinic visits. Therefore, their patient contacts include in-hospital services for clinic patients.

Chi-square analyses were used to compare recorded psychiatric diagnoses and psychotropic drug use among differing diagnostic, ethnic, and SES groups. Multiple logistic regression analysis was used to examine factors associated with the dichotomous dependent variables of psychiatric problems and psychotropic drug use.

RESULTS

Characteristics of the Sample

The majority of patients were male (96%) and with a mean age of 35 years (range: 17-63). Two hundred eighty-eight (64%) identified themselves as homosexual, 127 (22%) as bisexual, and 38 (8%) as heterosexual. One hundred seventeen (25%) of the patients were Hispanic and 71 (15%) were Black. One-half of the patients reported living with friends, 4% were living with a spouse, and 15% lived with other family members. A substantial number lived alone (24%). Few lived in community-sponsored housing (7%). In ranking patient occupations by the Duncan Socioeconomic Index (SEI) (Duncan, 1961), 41% of the patients fell in the lower, 32% in the middle, and 28% in higher socioeconomic status categories. Of the total population, 36% were able to continue employment.

The majority of patients (n = 247; 54%) had a diagnosis of ARC; one-third had AIDS (n = 180; 38%) and 35 of the patients (8%) were classified as minimally symptomatic. Ninety-seven patients had had *Pneumocystis carinii*, 75 had Kaposi's Sarcoma, and 18 had an organic CNS disorder. There were no significant differences in HIV diagnostic group by ethnicity or SES.

Risk Behavior Groups. Demographic and social characteristics did not vary by diagnostic group with the exception that there was a higher percentage of heterosexuals among the minimally symptomatic (χ^2 = 15.62, df4, p = .0001), and patients with AIDS were less likely to be employed (χ^2 = 17.06, df2, p = .001). Approximately one-fifth (n = 82) of the sample reported a history of intravenous (IV) drug use. (This percentage is consistent with Los Angeles data.) Intravenous drug use did not vary by diagnostic and SEI group, but did vary by ethnic group with (χ^2 = 26.75, df2, p = .01). Non-intravenous drug use was reported by almost 30% (n = 137) of the patients, with those most frequently reported being cocaine (n = 70) and marijuana (n = 62). Sixty-six patients reported current or past alcohol abuse, and 140 reported current or past alcohol use. Finally, the within-subject mean number of sexual partners reported for the years 1978-1986 declined substantially with time. The greatest decrease occurred between 1985, mean 15.37 and 1986, mean 6.62. Of special interest, this decline also occurred among self-reported drug users. Seventy-five patients reported having had sexual relations with a person with AIDS.

Mental Health Consultation. Only 7 patients (less than 1%) were seen by a psychiatric consultant. In each of these cases, the psychiatric problem was of such a severe nature that primary care staff required consultation. Two-hundred seventy-two patients (59%) were seen by one of the clinic social workers.

Psychiatric Problems

One hundred six, almost one-fourth of all patients, were reported to have a psychiatric diagnosis. Sixty-three of these patients were diagnosed as anxious during at least one clinic visit, and 37 as depressed. No patient was reported to be suicidal. It is noteworthy that the type and frequency of recorded psychiatric problems did not vary significantly among diagnostic and ethnic groups. However, significant variation by SEI was found, with depression most frequently diagnosed among upper SEI patients (χ^2 = 6.11, df2, p = < .05).

To examine whether demographic, social, and medical characteristics were associated with the presence of a psychiatric diagnosis, a logistic regression was conducted. Variables examined in the regression analysis included factors believed to predict or influence the recognition of psychological problems: diagnostic group, sexual preference, ethnicity, employment, IV drug use, and social isolation (Table 1). Controlling for all other variables, ethnicity was the only significant predictor. In particular, Anglos were more likely to have a psychiatric diagnosis than non-Anglos.

Psychotropic Drug Use

Eighty-nine patients (19%) were prescribed psychotropic medications during at least one clinic visit. The most frequently prescribed drugs were anti-anxiety agents (n = 59), anti-depressants (n = 29), and sedative-hypnotics (n = 26). No patient was prescribed an anti-psychotic medication. Psychotropic drug use varied significantly among AIDS, ARC, and minimally symptomatic patients (χ^2 = 8.71, df = 2, p = < .01). Of these groups, AIDS patients were most likely to be given psychotropic medication. This finding is noteworthy in view of the fact that psychiatric problems did not vary significantly among diagnostic groups. Psychotropic medication use did not vary by ethnic or SEI group. In fact, frequency of use among these groups was remarkably similar. Of those patients diagnosed with anxiety, 54% were prescribed psychotropic medications; of those with depression 59% and of those with any psychiatric diagnosis, 49% were given such drugs. In contrast, only 10% of the patients with no psychiatric diagnosis were prescribed psychotropic medications.

Logistic regression was also used to determine what factors predicted psychotropic medication use. The factors included HIV diag-

TABLE 1. Logistic Regression-Psychiatric Diagnosis

Variable	Parameter Estimate	χ^2	P
Diagnostic Group	−.19012	1.80	.1798
Sexual Preference	−.177671	1.71	.1909
Ethnicity	−.299599	4.73	.0297
Employment	−.232891	2.66	.1028
IV Drug	−.031046	0.04	.8483
Social Isolation	.139159	0.36	.5473

nostic group, sexual orientation, ethnicity, employment, diagnosis of psychiatric or CNS disorder, and social isolation (Table 2). For patients with either a psychiatric or CNS diagnosis, psychotropic medications were more likely to be prescribed. Even after controlling for other predictors, patients with AIDS were somewhat more likely to be given such medications.

Social Work Services

As previously noted, the majority of patients received clinic social work services. The minimally symptomatic were least likely to have been seen by a social worker (χ^2 = 13.75, df2, p = .001). Of those patients seen, almost all were assessed as having problems in adjusting to their illness. Surprisingly, only 28 (6%) were reported to have environmental problems such as financial, legal, or housing problems. AIDS patients were seen most frequently (χ^2 = 16.00, df4, p = .001). The majority of services provided involved individual counseling with patients. Social workers provided family counseling for 24% of the AIDS patients, 6% of ARC patients, and 9% of minimally symptomatic patients. A logistic regression was used to determine which factors were associated with whether a patient was seen by a social worker (Table 3). Patients with a

TABLE 2. Logistic Regression–Psychotropic Medications

Variable Parameter	Estimate	χ^2	p
Diagnostic Group	.267107	3.14	.0765
Sexual Preference	−.012357	0.01	.9344
Ethnicity	−.113068	0.53	.4668
Employment	−.135279	0.67	.4121
Psychiatric Diagnosis	.861113	31.71	.0001
CNS Diagnosis	.516624	4.13	.0422
Social Isolation	.039085	0.03	.8717

TABLE 3. Logistic Regression–Social Work Contact

Variable	Parameter Estimate	χ^2	p
Diagnostic Groups	.30289	6.91	.0086
Sexual Preference	−.025534	0.05	.8312
Ethnicity	−.163936	1.97	.1608
Employment	−.02614	0.05	.8293
Psychiatric Diagnosis	.462327	10.77	.0010
CNS Diagnosis	−.043675	0.03	.8649
Social Isolation	−.161002	0.53	.2083

psychiatric diagnosis and with AIDS were more likely to be seen by a clinic social worker.

DISCUSSION

This study is the first to document mental health service needs of an ambulatory, ethnoculturally diverse group of patients with not only AIDS, but also individuals with ARC and with minimal HIV-related symptoms. An appreciable number of patients within each of these three diagnostic groups were assessed by their primary care physician as having a psychiatric diagnosis and were prescribed at least one psychotropic medication. In addition, the majority of patients seen by social workers were assessed as having problems in adjusting to their illness. Noteworthy is the similar frequency of psychiatric and adjustment problems among patients in the three diagnostic groups suggesting that primary health care practitioners should routinely assess the psychological sequelae of patients with ARC and the minimally symptomatic as well those with AIDS. Data also suggest that future analyses of mental health services costs should include all persons with HIV-related illness (Harwood et al., 1984). Finally, study findings document the important role of primary medical care practitioners and social workers in providing mental health services to patients with HIV infections. Findings also suggest that psychiatric needs may be under-identified by primary care providers.

A comparison of the rate of psychiatric complications in the reported study with available data on patients with cancer and other medical conditions provides a context from which to view our study findings. Results from studies of hospitalized cancer patients using formal psychiatric evaluations generally report higher rates of psychiatric complications (up to nearly 50%) than those detected in the current study (Derogatis et al., 1983). In contrast, our findings more closely approximate those based on self-reported symptoms of depression among cancer patients (23%) (Plumb & Holland, 1977) and those found among general medical and primary practice populations, where rates range from 12% to 30%. Our finding that depression and anxiety were the most frequently diagnosed complications is similar to studies of cancer patients (Derogatis et al., 1983).

Of clinical import, comparisons with current published estimates of psychiatric problems among patients with HIV suggest that patient needs may be under-recognized by primary care physicians. On the other hand, the high percentage of patients evaluated by social workers in our study is noteworthy when compared to a recent study in which only 20% of all hospitalized cancer patients were referred for psychological and social services (Stam, Bultz, & Pittman, 1986). In this clinic, social workers are expected to provide mental health services. Therefore, it is likely that more formal psychiatric complications are diagnosed and treated under the broad recording category of adjustment problems. It is also likely that primary care physicians are relying, in part, on the clinic social workers to further evaluate patients' mental health needs.

Numerous and complex policy issues concerning primary prevention approaches to the HIV epidemic require immediate attention. At the same time, it is important that health care planning for providing care to those already ill is not neglected. The rapidly increasing numbers of patients with HIV infections entering the health care system increase the likelihood that many, if not most, patients will not be evaluated or cared for by a mental health practitioner, as was the case in our study. Given this caregiving context, health care planners must address two areas: the need for further research and for focused education programs for health professionals.

First, further studies are needed to identity risk factors for psychiatric complications of HIV infections. Once identified, such factors may be used to develop sensitive and specific assessment tools. Once these are developed, primary medical staff may be better trained to screen patients with HIV infection for mental health service need. Indeed, inexpensive screening mechanisms may improve the recognition rate of psychological problems by primary care physicians (Camerow, in press). Second, educational programs are needed to disseminate existing knowledge about the mental health needs of patients with HIV infections to primary health care practitioners.

Finally, our findings underscore the importance of taking into account the ethnocultural diversity of patients with HIV infections in future research and in educational programs. The finding that Anglo patients were more likely to have a psychiatric diagnosis than black and Hispanic patients raises the possibility that cultural influences may have masked recognition of psychiatric problems (Mays & Cochran, 1987). Similarly, failure to recognize depression among lower SES patients may have resulted from differences in communication styles between medical providers and lower SES patients (Frank, Eisenthal, & Lazare, 1978).

A discussion of study findings must be tempered by recognizing inherent limitations in a retrospective review of records. Furthermore, our findings may be applicable only to other groups of patients of similar ethnocultural and socioeconomic status such as those cared for at other large urban public hospitals. Finally, it must be remembered that knowledge concerning HIV illness is evolving very rapidly. At the time many of the study patients were receiving care, the CNS complications of the disease were not widely known. This may have contributed to under-reporting of mental health needs.

The vital role of primary health care practitioners, including social workers, in providing mental health services for patients with HIV infections is underscored by our results. Efforts to assist these practitioners in providing mental health services are undoubtedly an important area for immediate health policy planning.

REFERENCES

Baumgartner, G. (1985). *AIDS: Psychosocial Factors in the Acquired Immune Deficiency Syndrome*. Springfield, IL: Charles C. Thomas.

Belmont, M.F., Mantell, J.E. & Spivak, H.B. (1985). Resource utilization by AIDS patients in the acute care hospital. Final report summary submitted to the Health Services Improvement Fund, Inc. Empire Blue Cross/Blue Shield.

Burke, D.S., Brundage, J.F., Herbold, J.R., Berner, W., Gardner, L.I., Gunzenhauser, J.D., Voskivitch, J. & Redfield, R.R. (1987). Human Immunodeficiency Virus Infections among civilian applicants for United States Military Service, October 1985 to March 1986. *New England Journal of Medicine, 317*, 131-6.

Chase, M. AIDS costs: In lives and dollars. (May 18, 1987). *The Wall Street Journal*.

Christ, G. & Wiener, L. Psychosocial issues in AIDS. (1985). In *AIDS: Etiology, Diagnosis, Treatment and Prevention*, edited by V.T. Devita. Philadelphia: Lippincott.

Derogatis, L.R., Morrow, G.R., Fetting, J., Penman, D., Piasetsky, S., Schmale, A.M., Henrichs, M., & Carnicke, C.L.M. (1983). The prevalence of psychiatric disorders among cancer patients. *Journal of the American Medical Association, 249*, 751-57.

Detmer, W.M. Neuropsychiatric complications of AIDS: A literature review. (1986-87). *International Journal of Psychiatry in Medicine, 16*, 21-29.

Dilley, J.W., Ochitill, H.N., Per, M. & Volberding, P.A. (1985). Findings in psychiatric consultations with patients with Acquired Immune Deficiency Syndrome. *American Journal of Psychiatry, 142*, 82-86.

Duncan, O.D. A sociocultural index for all occupations. (1961). In *Occupations and Social Status*, edited by A.J. Reiss, Jr., O.D. Duncan, P.K. Hatt, & C.C. North. New York: Free Press.

Faulstich, M.E. (1987). Psychiatric aspects of AIDS. *American Journal of Psychiatry, 144*, 551-56.

Frank, A., Eisenthal, S. & Lazare, A. (1978). Are there social class differences in patients' treatment conceptions? *Archives of General Psychiatry, 35*, 61-69.

Goldberg, D. & Huxley, P. (1980). *Mental Illness in the Community*. London: Tavistock Publishing Company.

Hankin, J. & Oktay, J.S. (1979). *Mental disorders and primary medical care. An analytical review of the literature*. U.S. Government Printing Office. Pub. No. (ADM) 78-661: Washington, DC.

Harwood, H.J., Napolitano, D.M., Kristiansen, P.L., & Collins, J.J. (June, 1984). Economic costs to society of alcohol and drug abuse and mental illness: 1980. (Contract # ADM-283-83-0002) Research Park, NC: Research Triangle Institute, June, 1984.

Holland, J.C. & Tross S. (1985). The psychological and neuropsychiatric sequelae of the Acquired Immunodeficiency Syndrome and related disorders. *Annals of Internal Medicine, 103*, 760-764.

Institute of Medicine, National Academy of Sciences. (1986) *Confronting AIDS: Directions for Public Health, Health Care, and Research.* Washington, DC: National Academy Press.

Jaffe, H.W., Darrow, W.W., Echenberg, D.F., O'Malley P.M., Getchell, J.P., Kalyanarama, V.S., Byers, R.H., Drennan, D.P., Braff, E.H., and Curran, J.W. (1985). The Acquired Immunodeficiency Syndrome in a cohort of homosexual men: A six-year follow-up study. *Annals of Internal Medicine, 103,* 210-214.

Mays, V.M., & Cochran, S.D. (1987). Acquired Immunodeficiency Syndrome (AIDS) Black Americans: Social psychological issues. *Public Health Reports, 102,* 224-231.

Nichols, S.E. Jr. (1983). Psychiatric aspects of AIDS. *Psychosomatics, 24,* 1083-89.

Nurnberg, J., Prudic, J., Fiori, M. & Freedman, E. (1984). Psychopathology complicating Acquired Immune Deficiency Syndrome (AIDS). *American Journal of Psychiatry, 141,* 95-96.

Perry, S. & Jacobsen, P. (1986). Neuropsychiatric manifestations of AIDS-spectrum disorders. *Hospital and Community Psychiatry, 37,* 135-42.

Perry, S.W. & Markowitz, J. (1986). Psychiatric interventions for AIDS-spectrum disorders. *Hospital and Community Psychiatry, 37,* 1001-6.

Petty, F. & Noyes, R. (1981). Depression secondary to cancer. *Biological Psychiatry, 16,* 1203-20.

Plumb, M.M. & Holland, J. (1977). Comparative studies of psychosocial functions in patients with advanced cancer: I. Self-reported depressive symptoms. *Psychosomatic Medicine, 39,* 264-76.

Stam, H.J., Bultz, B.D., & Pittman, C.A. (1986). Psychosocial problems and interventions in a referred sample of cancer patients. *Psychomatic Medicine, 48,* 533-48.

Update: Acquired Immunodeficiency Syndrome in the San Francisco Cohort Study. (1985) *MMWR, 34,* 573-575.

Wolcott, D.L., Fawzy, F.I., & Pasnau, R.O. (1985). Acquired Immune Deficiency Syndrome (AIDS) and consultation-liaison psychiatry. *General Hospital Psychiatry, 7,* 280-292.

Wolcott, D.L., Fawzy, F., Landsverk, J., & McCombs, M. (1986). AIDS patients' needs for psychosocial services and their use of community service organizations. *Journal of Psychosocial Oncology, 4,* 135-46.

Chapter 7

The Use of Computerized
Need Projection Methodologies
to Implement Health Planning Policies

Jayasree Basu
Patricia A. Keimig

SUMMARY. Since 1982, the Maryland Health Resources Planning
Commission has developed a substantial proportion of its planning
effort to the development of need projection methodologies that
fulfill the policy direction established in the State Health Plan. Because each service, for which need is projected, has a unique set of
problems, policy direction leads to service-specific approaches to
forecasting need. Each methodology takes into consideration appropriate minimum sizes and distribution of services, rates of
growth, and reallocation of use from overserved to underserved
areas. Examples from acute medical/surgical, acute psychiatric,
comprehensive rehabilitation, and institutional long-term care services are given.

INTRODUCTION

Maryland's approach to problems in health care delivery, particularly those related to cost and access to care, includes extensive use
of regulation. It was the fourth state in the nation to enact a certificate of need program and one of the first to institute statewide
mandatory rate-setting for hospitals. It is one of only two states

This chapter was originally published in *Journal of Health & Social Policy*, Vol.
2(2) 1990.

maintaining an all-payor rate-setting system following enactment of the Medicare Prospective Payment System. Although a number of services have been removed from certificate of need review in recent years (end-stage renal disease treatment facilities, domiciliary care, and, most significantly, major medical equipment), regulation of other services has been strengthened (ambulatory surgical facilities, and drug abuse treatment facilities). Major medical equipment is now subject to licensure to assure quality of care, and utilization review is required for all hospital patients.

Since its creation in 1982, the Maryland Health Resources Planning Commission–the successor to earlier statewide health planning agencies dating back to the late 1960s–has devoted a considerable portion of its planning effort to developing better methods of forecasting need for regulated services. This paper explains, using four of the commission's current need projection methodologies, the ways in which computer technology is used to carry out commission policies and enhance its ability to forecast need.

Forecasted need for specific services is used in certificate of need review to carry out commission policies of orderly growth to meet statewide need, prohibition of growth and orderly reductions in areas of excess, and allocation or reallocation of services to areas of greater relative need. In each case, forecasting need is a balance among considerations of cost, access, and quality of care, and the final result is a combination of policy judgment and complex methodological steps aided by computer technology.

Forecasting the future involves improving the accuracy of what is, in essence, a crystal ball. However, sustained effort in this field, as in any other, tends to narrow the range of error. The most time-honored methods of doing so involve improving the data base, taking into account more variables, and increasing the statistical sophistication of forecasting techniques.

DATA SETS

Forecasting is only as good as the data available. Four types of data are used by the commission in forecasting need: (1) population estimates and projections, (2) inventories of services, (3) utilization data, and (4) national studies and data. The commission's efforts have focused on the latter three, since other state agencies are responsible, under Maryland law, for developing population estimates and projections. Estimates and projections are available for five year cohorts by sex and race (white and nonwhite) for each county for each year through 1995. Projections for the years 2000 and 2010 are also available. Out-of-state population data provided by the U.S. Bureau of the Census or other state agencies are also used. The commission's efforts with respect to population data have primarily assured that only one source of data may legally be used, and that conflicting claims about population estimates and projections do not reduce the credibility of its forecasts.

Development and maintenance of inventories of existing services have become, over time, tasks carried out largely by the commission. While state licensure records provide the basis for many inventories, they have proved to be inadequately detailed and, in addition, are not published in a usable form. For example, records of licensed hospital beds by service are not uniform from hospital to hospital. The commission now maintains inventories of the following services: acute medical-surgical, pediatric, obstetrical, and psychiatric beds; nursing home beds; intermediate care beds for alcohol and drug abuse treatment; residential treatment center beds for mentally ill children and adolescents; long-term psychiatric care beds; chronic disease beds; ambulatory surgical facilities; comprehensive rehabilitation beds; home health and hospice agencies; and organized primary care services.

Collection and analysis of Maryland utilization data have also become major data activities of the commission. These are the primary sources of data for determining need, where appropriate and available. Among the Maryland facilities surveyed by the commission are nursing homes, home health agencies, hospices, cardiac surgical and catheterization facilities, and freestanding ambulatory surgical facilities. The commission works with other agencies to collect data from hospitals, psychiatric facilities, and alcohol and drug abuse treatment facilities. Much remains to be done to assure an adequate amount of utilization data on health care services.

When Maryland data are unavailable or inappropriate, the commission relies on national studies and data. For example, Maryland data on acute psychiatric utilization, although available, are not used as they inadequately reflect the need for services. National estimates are used instead, and are adjusted to adapt them to Maryland's situation. National data are consulted for comparative purposes even when Maryland data are considered complete and reliable. Trends in acute care admissions at the national level, and comparisons between states under the Medicare Prospective Payment System (PPS) and non-PPS states, are examples of important data used in forecasting statewide admissions and length of stay variables.

METHODS

State of the art techniques for forecasting bed need can be characterized as utilization methods, simulation methods, and statistical distribution methods. Those used by the commission at present are, for the most part, utilization methods. The advantages of utilization methods are their relative simplicity, understandability, and adaptability to service-specific data. In addition, standards can be established that relate directly to variables used, such as occupancy.[1]

Good data for all services are still insufficient to allow the commission to develop and test comprehensive simulation models.[2] Statistical distribution approaches view admissions and discharges as random events and bed need as an expression of a predetermined probability that a patient will be turned away a given percent of the time. This kind of approach is partially used by the commission for acute obstetrical services. While statistical distribution methods can be appropriate for institutional planning, there are difficulties in adapting them for regional planning that covers more than one facility. Furthermore, they are by definition demand-based and are therefore unsuited to services for which demand may not be a good indicator of need.[3] Neither simulation nor statistical distribution methods are discussed in this chapter, so our focus is on the commission's use of utilization methods.

When we take the oldest existing utilization formula for determining bed need, we are looking at the bed-to-population ratio developed for use in the Hill-Burton hospital construction program, that existed from 1946 through the early 1970s. The formula can be written thus:

$$NEED = (RATIO)(POP), \tag{1}$$

where NEED is bed need, RATIO is beds per population, and POP is population. The ratio was set, at various times and for various places, between 4.0 and 5.5 beds per 1,000 population; figures that nearly everyone today agrees are too high.

Unfortunately, this formula can convey little information about one community's need for beds in relation to another's with respect to differences in demographic structure, socioeconomic and health status, medical practice patterns, distance from other available sources of care, and use of other facilities. New variables, however, can be created from this simple formula to make it better suited to capture these differences. Equation (1) can be rewritten thus:

$$NEED = \frac{DAYS,}{(365)(OCC)} \tag{2}$$

where DAYS is patient days, and OCC is occupancy. A refinement of the DAYS variable produces:

$$NEED = \frac{(ADM)\ (ALOS),}{(365)(OCC)} \tag{3}$$

where ADM is admissions or discharges, and ALOS is average length of stay.

Equations (2) and (3) offer the primary variables used by the commission in most of its projections for hospitals and other types of beds, but still do not speak to variations by age, sex, race, diagnosis, payor group, place of residence, and place of care. These disaggregations of the primary variables dramatically improve the relevance and usefulness of a utilization-based method, while also increasing the dependence of need projections on computer technology.

The models used by the commission for forecasting the future values of these variables are essentially deterministic in nature. The main reasons that structural models are not used, are the wide diversity of factors that influence these variables and the present inability to capture all these influences adequately in a structural model.

The remainder of this paper presents the ways computer technology is important to the commission in projecting need. The value of computer technology is evident in three ways:

(1) Using large data sets, developing a baseline projection that:

    a. calculates base-year rates of admission, average lengths of stay, and rates of patient days for a multi-dimensional array of age groups, payor groups, geographic areas of origin (that includes out-of-state areas), and services; and

    b. identifies the migration pattern of patients from areas of origin to areas of care in Maryland (usually counties), and forecasts need in counties on the basis of the base-year utilization pattern;

(2) Carrying out complex modifications of use rates, lengths of stay, and migration patterns to tailor the results to account for differences in communities and to reflect policy goals; and

(3) Preparing supplementary data analyses.

We discuss service-specific need methodologies for four services to illustrate how the variables presented in equations (2) and (3) are manipulated by computer to arrive at need projection models that carry out commission policies. Each methodology differs in terms of its approach to forecasting need. In the following section, we discuss these approaches in a general way before presenting detailed examples.

APPROACHES TO FORECASTING NEED

Most acute care services exist in sufficient or excess amounts in Maryland. The commission's general policies for most acute care services are to prohibit statewide growth and to selectively encourage growth only in counties with rapid population increases. A demand-based approach, which uses Maryland admission rates and lengths of stay, is appropriate since utilization is not constrained by the supply of services but only by effective demand. The problem lies in identifying future trends in an era of unstable trends that are poor predictors of future demand. The commission uses a variety of analyses to arrive at statewide values and then distributes them in predetermined ways to alter each county's initial projections consistent with the statewide values.

In long-term care, statewide use rates by age (demand), measured by patient days, are considered to be a reasonable overall indicator of need in Maryland, particularly since neither waiting lists for admission to nursing homes nor administrative days in hospitals awaiting placement in nursing homes are salient issues at the present time (although waiting lists and difficult-to-place patients are important issues in some counties). The general policies are controlled growth statewide and allocating growth to assure that proportionately more beds are built in counties with low use rates and high out-migration, thus assuring services nearer to home. The problem is finding the best way to allocate new beds when not enough is known about the causes of community differences in use rates and without enough years of good data to undertake trend analysis. The commission starts with county use rates, but adjusts these in such a way as to redistribute services to each county so that use rates approach the statewide mean more closely. The commission also reallocates patient days by making upward adjustments in the retention rates of each county in a manner discussed later in this chapter.

Comprehensive rehabilitation services, unlike either acute or long-term care, are in low supply and low demand. For this service, the general policies create more services statewide and assure an even distribution of services to each region. The problem here is identification of an appropriate measure of need. Lacking Maryland data for rehabilitation care, the commission starts with Maryland acute care utilization and forecasts, and through a series of ratios for each diagnosis code and population group (established by expert opinion), figures the number of admissions that can be expected to need inpatient rehabilitation following an acute care stay. Lengths of stay are derived from the national data on rehabilitation hospitals since Maryland data are unavailable.

Acute psychiatric care, like comprehensive rehabilitation services, is inadequate statewide and is unevenly distributed regionally. A large amount of unmet need is believed to exist. Here utilization is a result of both inadequate supply and low demand and utilization cannot be taken as a measure of need. The policies create more services statewide and focus most of the growth in the most poorly served regions. The problem, again, is identification of an appropriate indicator of need. A demand-based methodology employing Maryland use rates would be inappropriate. The commission, therefore, begins by looking at national prevalence rates derived from research and then adjusts for local factors. Lengths of stay are derived from Maryland data on psychiatric admissions.

In the next two sections of the chapter we discuss baseline projections and how to tailor those projections for three of the services we have already introduced. Because the commission's approach to acute psychiatric services does not involve a baseline projection, it is discussed later in the chapter.

BASELINE PROJECTIONS

Each of the three projections that begins with base-year utilization is derived through a complex set of mathematical steps, and shares several common elements. These complex mathematical steps are performed on very large data bases, and involve substantial use of computer technology and programming capability. The common steps result in a baseline projection in which utilization is projected in each area of care in Maryland. This projection is based on rates of patient days or discharges in the base year in each age group by the residents of each jurisdiction (counties and other states), who are admitted to facilities in the county of care, and population changes from the base to the target year in the corresponding age group and jurisdiction of residence. It can be expressed in the following general equations:

$$TU_{ijk} = (BU_{ijk})(POPCH_{ik}), \text{ and} \qquad (4)$$

$$TU_j = \underset{i\,k}{TU_{ijk}} \qquad (5)$$

where TU is target year utilization, BU is base year utilization (discharges or patient days), POPCH is the population change ratio, "i" is jurisdiction of residence (Maryland counties and out of state), "j" is county of care in Maryland, and "k" is age group.

Equation (4) projects target year utilization on the basis of two assumptions: (a) utilization will grow at the same rate as the population in each age group from base to the target year in each county from which patients are coming; and (b) patient migration patterns from jurisdiction of origin to county of care will remain the same from base to target year.

Equations (4) and (5) determine the basic nature of the baseline projection for each of the three projection methodologies. However, different levels of disaggregation are used for each service. In acute care, equation (4) is further disaggregated by service, determined by groups of diagnosis related categories (DRGs), and by age. In addition, discharges and average lengths of stay are initially projected separately for each county, using constant use rates for both discharges and patient days (used to obtain lengths of stay) from the base to target year. In long-term care, on the other hand, equations (4) and (5) are not disaggregated further and discharges and average lengths of stay are merged into a single patient day variable. The baseline projection is not explicitly made because adjustments in use rates and migration are made in this methodology simultaneously with setting up the initial projection. We discuss this later in the chapter.

Projecting need for comprehensive rehabilitation services is done using the most complex of the commission's methodologies in terms of its computer orientation and technology-intensiveness. This methodology projects discharges and average lengths of stay separately. Average lengths of stay are derived from national rehabilitation hospital data, disaggregated by age and diagnosis group.[4] The projection of discharges is done using the same assumptions as involved in equation (4). However, equation (4) is further disaggregated by diagnosis or procedure. The multi-dimensional matrix represents, for each patient, age group, jurisdiction of origin, area of care, and diagnosis (primary and secondary) or procedure at the ICD-9 level. Proportions are used for each diagnosis or procedure to represent need for rehabilitation services. The number of patients discharged with each diagnosis or procedure in each age group from each jurisdiction of residence are multiplied by these proportions. The diagnosis and procedure codes included in the methodology, and the proportions used, are based on the judgment of Maryland experts in rehabilitation services. The hundreds of primary and secondary diagnosis and procedure codes, together with other analytical details such as age-adjustment, make the scope of this methodology much greater than others we know of for this service.[5]

In order to illustrate the complexity of this methodology, parameters that are estimated in the methodology by computer are presented:

$$RADM_{ikjd} = (AADM_{ikjd})(PCT_{jd}), \qquad (6)$$

there $RADM_{ikjd}$ is the number of rehabilitation admissions expected to be generated by residents of area "i" in age group "k" who were hospitalized in area "j" with a diagnosis or procedure code "d" in the base year; $AADM_{ikjd}$ is the number of residents of area "i" in age group "k" who are admitted in acute care hospitals in area "j" with diagnosis or procedure code "d" in the base year; and PCT_{jd} is the estimated proportion of patients hospitalized in area "j" with diagnosis or procedure code "d" in the base year.

Then,

$$TDAYS_{ikjd} = (RADM_{ikjd})(POPCH_{ik})(ALOS_{jkd}), \qquad (7)$$

where $TDAYS_{ikjd}$ is the number of patient days which are expected to be generated by residents of area "i" in age group "k" who are hospitalized in area "j" with diagnosis or procedure code "d" in the target year; $POPCH_{ik}$ is the proportional change in population in area "i" in age group "k" from base to the target year; and $ALOS_{jkd}$ is the desired average length of stay for patients in area "j" in age group "k" with diagnosis code "d."

Patient days for area j are finally projected as:

$$TDAYS_j = \sum_{i=1}^{32} \sum_{k=1}^{6} \sum_{d=1}^{n} TADAYS_{ikjd} \qquad (8)$$

Equations (7) and (8) are variations of equations (4) and (5) at higher levels of disaggregation. In order to carry out these calculations, a mainframe computer is used as it can deal with large data sets and complex multi-dimensional matrices efficiently. It is implemented by use of high-level programming skills to make its timely production possible.

One of the primary components in developing baseline projections for each area is accounting for the migration behavior of patients. Measuring migration requires collecting patient-specific utilization data by the resident county (or state) and, sometimes, zip code. Within-state migration and migration from other states can be accounted for with these data. Migration out of state, which is a significant number of all patient days in many states like Maryland, is considerably tougher to ascertain, and the commission has not always been successful since surrounding states do not have comparable data. For this reason, the "true" patient use rates and retention rates are unknown in many Maryland counties. Therefore the commission's need forecasts do not attempt to use them.

The reasons for migration cannot be identified without data collection currently beyond the resources of the commission. Migration can occur for many reasons. Those that are important include local maldistribution of services of which there may be an adequate supply statewide, and poor-quality or difficult-to-access services that cause people to obtain care elsewhere. The first is addressed directly in the need projection while the second is addressed in standards used to govern the commission's certificate of need program. Other reasons for migration are generally caused by either genuine "patient choice" (which includes physician preference) or migration to regional or specialized services, that are looked upon by the commission as legitimate reasons for migration that should be protected when forecasting need.

TAILORING BASELINE PROJECTIONS

The baseline projections for two of the services discussed in the last section are modified in different ways to meet different policy concerns. These modifications are discussed in this section.

Acute care discharges and average lengths of stay are separately projected by service (pediatric, obstetrical, and medical/surgical/ gynecological/addictions). This data is subdivided further into payor groups: Medicare, Medicaid, Blue Cross, and Other. (Initial need for obstetrical services is not calculated using the baseline need projection technique, but instead is based on the expected number of live births and other factors determining obstetrical admissions.)

Once the initial projection is completed, adjustments are made in both projected average lengths of stay and projected admissions. Statewide expected values for the target year are determined for each service and payor group through a series of trend analyses, including linear and nonlinear regressions. Use of these analytic methods to help establish these values is discussed later in this chapter.

Target average lengths of stay for each county are established by making adjustments that reflect the difference between the state-wide initial projection, that use base-year use rates applied to the target year population, and the expected value in the target year, derived from a combination of data analysis and expert judgment. Differences in length of stay between base year total and county average length of stay is taken into account. The average length of stay for each county is derived by using each hospital's case mix with a mean average length of stay, which creates a county-weighted average length of stay. The method of doing these adjustments can be shown as follows:

$$ADTLOS_j = TLOS_j - (DCLOS + CM_j)(TLOS_j), \qquad (9)$$

where ADTLOS is adjusted target year length of stay, TLOS is the average length of stay initially projected in the target year, DCLOS is the proportional statewide change in average length of stay from projected to targeted value, CM are the differences in county length of stay between the actual and the case-mix adjusted length of stay, and j is the county of utilization. A floor is established below which county target lengths of stay are not permitted to fall.

This procedure results in narrowing differences in county average lengths of stay that cannot be explained by case-mix differences, and also carries out commission policy to project reductions in statewide average lengths of stay to at least the national average.[6]

Target admissions (for each county are projected by establishing expected statewide admission values for each service and payor group and proportionately adjusting the county's projected admissions to arrive at the expected total. This step ensures that the initial projection based on constant use rates by age is modified in relation to not only the statewide expected value but to each county's use rate in the base year, resulting in variations from baseline use rates to targeted use rates for each service and payor group. As in target county lengths of stay, the range of variation in the admission rate among the counties is narrowed, but unlike the length of stay adjustments, the differences are not narrowed around a predetermined mean (the statewide expected length of stay) but are narrowed in relation to the predetermined new total (the statewide expected admissions). Consequently, the adjustment fulfills the commission's policy to project reductions in variations in admissions per capita for given diagnoses among small areas in Maryland[7] and is consistent with literature suggesting that small-area variations in rates of admission are larger than community differences suggest is necessary.[8]

The long-term care methodology uses patient days as the basic variable. Unlike acute care, where use rate adjustments to the initial projection are made in subsequent steps, the long-term care methodology has a built-in adjustment mechanism in the initial projection itself. In projecting target use rates by county, the base year use rates are normalized and then altered to bring outliers closer to the statewide mean. This procedure modifies extreme variations in use rates.

Also unlike acute care or rehabilitation services–for which the base year migration pattern is projected onto the target year–the long-term care methodology adjusts retention by returning half the patient days expected to be incurred outside the county of residence back to the county. This results in a one-to-one reduction in the patient days from each county where in-migration occurs. This step is carried out to implement the commission's policy to correct the maldistribution of services and increase the retention rate of each county.[9]

In reviewing methodologies used in other states, we found that, while many use local use rates, adjustments in these rates are most often based on assumptions regarding unnecessary days in nursing homes and administrative days in hospitals. Few states seem to use migration data to return days to communities of origin.[10]

ACUTE PSYCHIATRIC SERVICES

The last example that we discuss in this paper is the projection of acute psychiatric services, that is unique in terms of its approach to the need projection problem, although it is less dependent on computer technology. National estimated prevalence rates by age groups are used for projecting statewide need, while local need is projected on the basis of socio-demographic differences in different areas of the state. Maryland's approach to forecasting need for this service differs from that of other health planning agencies that use socio-demographic indicators by being the first, to our knowledge, to have translated these indicators into bed need estimates through a causal relationship discussed later.[11]

The steps used are as follows:

(1) An estimate of uniform prevalence is made using the projected population and national projected prevalence rates by age groups derived from the Graduate Medical Education National Advisory Committee (GMENAC) study.[13]

(2) Socio-demographic differences among counties are accounted for by the application of a composite score value (Z-score) indicating socio-demographic need of those areas. This Z-score is derived by using selected variables derived from National Institute of Mental Health's 1980 *Demographic Profile Tape* and other Maryland-specific demographic data. The variables were screened for their demonstrated usefulness in previous research, comparability, stability over the long run, and statistical independence from each other. The six social indicators chosen were the percent of: minority population, persons in poverty, divorced persons, school dropouts, widowed females, and persons receiving public assistance. A composite score value of these indicators was estimated by transforming these variables into Z values and averaging them.

(3) A relationship is established to convert the Z values into population-in-need estimates. This relationship was derived from current research on mental health need assessment[13] and can be expressed as:

$$NPOP = PRE(1 + 0.2Z), \tag{10}$$

where NPOP is the population in need, PRE is uniform prevalence, and Z is the Z-score. The rationale for using a parameter value (0.2) is explained in other studies.[14] Such a parameter value can produce a range of prevalence rates between areas of about 2-to-1, which was an acceptable range according to epidemiological data available when the projection was made.

(4) The population in need estimate derived in step (3) is converted into estimates of required acute care admissions and beds by using the following steps:

a. Using GMENAC assumptions about intervention rates by service settings in two age groups (children/adolescents and adults), the number of required acute admissions for Maryland residents in two age groups is determined.

b. Adjustments are made for migration to other states and in-migration of out-of-state residents to Maryland.

c. Further adjustments are made for expected migration between planning regions by assuming that a proportion of existing migration can be attributed to patient choice.

d. Statewide average lengths of stay for each age group are projected forward and used for determining each area's bed need.

These steps carry out the policies of estimating unmet need, particularly in communities wholly without acute psychiatric services, and addressing the maldistribution of beds throughout the state.[15]

It is of interest to note that the commission's basic approach was used in a subsequent study contracted for by the Maryland Mental Hygiene Administration to estimate need for acute and other psychiatric services. While the study differed from the commission's approach in its length of stay value, in using episodes rather than individuals as the unit of projection, and in counting as acute additional beds in private psychiatric hospitals, it explicitly adopted the commission's method of establishing socio-demographic composite values and converting them to bed need estimates.[16]

SUPPLEMENTARY DATA ANALYSES

While the computer is necessary for the manipulation of large data sets and calculations using multi-dimensional matrices needed to compute need projections, it is also essential in undertaking data analyses that assist development of the methodology or of key variables in a given methodology. We discuss a few types of analyses in this section.

Trend analysis is used to evaluate trends in acute care discharges and average length stay for Maryland hospitals, for which there is a data set complete enough, good enough, and with enough years (1979 forward) to permit time-series analysis. Trends in admissions at both the major diagnosis code level (24 groups) and diagnosis related group level (467 groups) have been evaluated. Data for case mix-adjusted average length of stay, case mix, and actual length of stay have been compared to identify how actual length of stay has varied over time in relation to changes in case mix and changes in case mix-adjusted average length of stay. A detailed analysis of these factors, together with comparisons with national trends, has helped to establish key statewide values in acute care.

Regression analysis was used in preliminary evaluation of a proposed demand-based acute psychiatric services model. A variety of socio-demographic indicators were used in a stepwise multiple regression model relating these indicators to current utilization of acute psychiatric services in Maryland by area to identify significant variables determining need for mental health care. This regression contributed to the decision to abandon a demand-based approach in favor of the one described in this chapter.

Correlation analysis was used in developing the acute psychiatric model described above to evaluate the importance of local sociodemographic factors identifying populations at risk for mental illness. About 30 such indicators were tested for their usefulness in predicting mental health need. Their relationships with each other were evaluated by a correlation matrix in order to eliminate the use of indicators that correlate with each other very highly.

Case-mix adjustment was used in developing the acute care projection in two ways. First, trends in the statewide case mix-adjusted average length of stay were evaluated and compared to the national trend. The commission's staff has developed special programs to automate the computation of a case-mix index for Maryland. Second, the county actual average length of stay was compared to the case mix-adjusted length of stay and adjustment was made for their differences in computing the targeted ALOS. Both methods of case-mix adjustment depend on a computer sort of discharge data for each patient by diagnosis related group and payor to use them in the case-mix adjustment model.

In the next section, we briefly present some of the applications of need projections in decisions made by the commission in its certificate of need programs, and some general effects of need projections on industry behavior.

USES AND EFFECTS

The commission has created a variety of decision-making tools within its certificate of need program. Each of these tools uses the need projection in a different way.

In uncontested, single-applicant reviews, need projections act as ceilings for approval of the projected number of beds or services. An applicant is not permitted to request approval for beds projected to be needed in areas outside its own, generally a county or defined group of counties.

The need projection is also used as ceiling for batched, multiapplicant reviews. In these types of reviews, the need projection can affect the number of applicants approved. A possible result is approval of fewer beds than the projection allows if the best projects do not collectively apply for all the beds forecasted to be needed. This can result in a second round of applications, but it is more likely that applicants will modify their existing applications upward or that existing facilities will "use up" the remaining allowable beds in small non-reviewable bed additions.

In some instances, a new need projection becomes effective in the midst of a certificate of need review. In most cases, applicants must modify their applications downward if fewer beds are projected to be needed, and may modify upward if more are expected to be needed. For nursing home batches, which are often quite large, a special rule fixing the effective projection, after applications are accepted for review but before administrative hearings are held, is included in the state health plan. This rule provides some predictability in the largest single arena in which the commission undertakes time-consuming batched reviews.

Finally, the need projection can be used to arrive at a "summary" certificate of need decision to deny an application. If an applicant applies for beds in a county for which none are projected to be needed, the commission can simply establish this in a brief decision that does not rely on other aspects of the applicant's proposal.

In addition to the specific decisions made by the commission in certificate of need reviews, its need projection affects and alters the behavior of the industry. Few applications are even received in areas of no need or excess capacity. This has permitted a partial deregulation of hospitals by allowing each facility to annually configure its medical/surgical, pediatric, and obstetrical beds in the amount it perceives to be most appropriate, provided the total bed complement of all three services does not increase. The reasoning behind this change in the commission's statute lay in the general excess of beds in each of these three services in most counties in the state. The exact size of the excess in each service then becomes relatively unimportant.

Another general effect is the support the need projection gives to Maryland's statewide, all-payor utilization control mechanism. Effective utilization control, required by statute in 1985, partially depends upon constraints in available beds to work. This is the converse of Roemer's Law: "A bed built is a bed filled is a bed billed."

It is generally acknowledged that certificate of need is designed to replace, in important respects, market competition in the construction and enlargement of health care facilities. Need projections adopted by the commission enhance these effects since applicants do not have an opportunity to prove need on their own. There are two consequences to this result. First, the commission focuses its decisions on questions of financial access to care, optimum cost and quality of care, and uses the certificate of need program to foster a variety of policy goals. This is similar to the effects of constraining the supply of physicians in order to raise the quality of the physician pool above that likely to be produced if physicians were not licensed.

Second, the commission can assure a better distribution of facilities than that likely to be produced if certificate of need did not channel development. For each area of the state, a need projection makes beds possible and unavailable for approval elsewhere. This is the commission's chief means of improving geographic access to services.

CONCLUSION

In this chapter, we discussed the individual nature of need projection methodologies now in use in Maryland. Because of very large patient-specific data bases, and the separate nature of each approach, these methodologies are computerized to the extent possible and to the extent that it is efficient to do so. In some cases, such as in the case of comprehensive rehabilitation services, the methodology is calculated entirely on a mainframe computer, because the capabilities of micro- and mini-computers are insufficient. For others, a combination of mainframe and microcomputers is used for the data handling process. Regardless of the way the need projection is done, it is used to carry out the commission's mission to ensure equal access to quality health care at a reasonable cost by its role in certificate of need decisions and effect on individual investment decisions made by existing and would-be health care facilities.

REFERENCE NOTES

1. B.Z. Palmer. Methods, Standards, and Data for Areawide Acute Care Hospital Planning. Bethesda, MD: Alpha Center, June 1982.

2. Ibid.

3. Ibid.

4. Hospital Utilization Project: Rehabilitation Facility Program for 1984 Data. Later data are used when the projection is updated.

5. Alpha Center: Update. July 1983; Based on a survey of other states, the closest to the commission's is the Physical Rehabilitation Services Plan in the 1982-87 New Jersey State Health Plan.

6. State Health Plan: Acute Inpatient Services. Maryland COMAR 10.24.10, effective February 8,1988.

7. Ibid.

8. Division of Medical Practice Patterns: Variations in the Use of Medical and Surgical Services by the Maryland Population. Baltimore, MD: Maryland Department of Health and Mental Hygiene, December 1986; J.E. Wennberg and A.M. Gittelsohn. A Small Area Approach to the Analysis of Health System Perfor-

mance. Final Report, HRA contract no. 291-76-0003. Hyattsville, MD: Health Resources Administration, 1980.

9. Maryland State Health Plan. Maryland COMAR 10.24.07, Supplement 5, effective December 15, 1986.

10. J.M. Walsh. A Compendium of Substantive Methodologies from the Plan Documents File. Prepared under contract no. HRA-232-79-0037. Washington, DC: U.S. Department of Health and Human Services, April 1986.

11. Ibid; M.R. Isaacs. Acute Psychiatric Bed Need Planning: Issues and Methodologies. Methodological Note No. 6, U.S. Department of Health and Human Services, February 1986.

12. Office of Graduate Medical Education, Health Resources Administration: Physician Requirements–1990 for Psychiatry. Rockville, MD: U.S. Department of Health and Human Services, May 1981.

13. R.E. Grosser. A Model to Estimate Population in Need of Mental Health Services by Catchment Area. Colorado Division of Mental Health. Presented at The Third National Conference on Need Assessment in Health and Human Service Systems, March 17-20, 1981, Louisville, Kentucky.

14. Ibid.

15. Maryland State Health Plan: Maryland COMAR 10.24.07, Supplement 6, effective February 9, 1987.

16. H.H. Goldman, K. Marvelle, M.S. Ridgely, and M. Gabay. Study of Statewide Inpatient Mental Health Services, Maryland Mental Hygiene Administration. Final contract report, June 22, 1987.

Chapter 8

Psychosocial Factors as Predictors of Length of Stay of Medicare Patients Under the Prospective Payment System

Barry Rock
Marian Goldstein
Marybeth Hopkins
Elizabeth B. Quitkin

SUMMARY. The Prospective Payment System methodology is designed to predict inpatient hospital resource utilization. The system sets standards based on medical diagnosis (Diagnosis Related Groups), but it ignores psychosocial characteristics which often determine discharge options and therefore, directly affect a patient's length of stay. A study is described which examined the psychosocial characteristics of 234 elderly hospitalized patients in relation to length of stay and route of admission (elective or emergency room). Such data can be very useful to discharge planners in identifying high social risk patients, as well as to health planners attempting to modify the DRG methodology to incorporate psychosocial factors.

INTRODUCTION

The prospective payment system (PPS) utilizing diagnostic related groups (DRGs), a form of health care rationing, (Aaron & Schwartz, 1984) has placed considerable pressures on hospitals for

This chapter was originally published in *Journal of Health & Social Policy*, Vol. 2(2) 1990.

rapid discharge of elderly patients (Caputi & Heiss, 1984; Patchner & Wattenberg, 1985; Reamer, 1985; Wolock & Schlesinger, 1986). Recent efforts to revise health care financing in the United States have involved rationing only, and in the absence of a comprehensive health care policy issues of quality, access, and equity have largely been ignored (Rock, 1987). PPS is a form of capitation in which payments for hospital care of the elderly under Medicare are flat fees based on diagnosis (DRGs) and are not related to actual costs or actual length of stay (LOS). Thus, there is an incentive for hospitals to discharge patients as soon as it is medically appropriate (and hopefully not before).

Psychosocial problems, especially those related to post-hospital care, often contribute to longer lengths of stay. In many hospitals, departments of social work are perceived as having the expertise to cut costs by providing effective discharge planning services to patients and families (Schrager et al., 1978; Vielhaber & Irwin, 1975). Timely and comprehensive discharge planning for patients' post-hospital care is a critical component of efforts to minimize the need for protracted inpatient hospital stays (Boone, Coulton, & Keller, 1981; Coulton et al., 1982; Glass & Weiner, 1976; Herman, Culpepper, & Franks, 1984; Rossen & Colton, 1985).

The research of Berkman and Rehr on the critical significance of the timing of medical social work intervention in promoting effective discharge planning further emphasizes the importance of addressing this issue. Their analysis of a series of studies in the early 1970s and 1980s revealed that the timing of intervention most often occurred "between the second and third weeks of hospitalization rather than immediately after admission, the crucial period for the patient and family" (Berkman & Rehr, 1970). In a subsequent study, the authors developed a framework for the "sick-role cycle," identifying five stages of the patient experience: (1) the symptom experience phase (2) the assumption of the sick role (3) the medical care contact stage (4) the dependent patient phase, and (5) the recovery phase (Berkman & Rehr, 1972). Referrals to hospital social work services usually involved the latter two phases in which patients encounter stress in assuming the dependent patient role and in which there are, ". . . a predominance of social needs related to the post-hospital phase of patient care" (Berkman & Rehr, 1972,

p. 573). Most of the cases in the study had been referred to social work in the "recovery phase," not allowing intervention in the earlier stages in which psychosocial adjustment of patient and family to illness and hospitalization took place; in this last stage, it was often too late for effective discharge planning.

In contrast, in the third study of the series, the traditional method of referrals was contrasted with one in which social workers controlled their own early case finding. As might be anticipated, "it was found that under independent case finding, social workers. . . reach significantly more patients and family members early in the course of hospitalization and . . . reach considerably more persons in need of help related to being ill. . ." (Berkman & Rehr, 1973, p. 256). Having established the efficacy of social work controlled case finding and early intervention, later articles have focused on techniques for screening and identification of patients with high social risk profiles (Berkman, Rehr, & Rosenberg, 1980).

In recognition of social work's crucial role in discharge planning, and in an effort to improve workers' ability to develop appropriate plans which will facilitate timely hospital releases, a number of hospital social work departments have instituted programs of case finding, high-risk screening, early intervention, and pre-admission programs (Berkman et al., 1988; Reardon et al., 1988).

STUDY

The Long Island Jewish Medical Center is a multi-campus urban/suburban teaching hospital located in New Hyde Park, New York. The Long Island Jewish (LIJ) division has 342 medical/surgical beds. While an average of 32 percent of the patients in the hospital at any given time are 65 years-of-age or over, 48 percent of patient days are Medicare.

With the implementation of the Federal Prospective Payment System in New York State on January 1, 1986, concern grew about managing lengths of stay for elderly patients at the medical center. The Social Work Department in particular focused its attention on this issue. In a 1981 study conducted at LIJ, 40 percent of all social work cases were opened in the first week of a patient's stay, and an additional 30 percent were opened in the second week. At that time, it was considered admirable that 70 percent of all cases were opened by the fourteenth day. With the implementation of DRGs, however, this result was considered intolerable. Consideration was given to the development of an early intervention system which would allow high-risk cases to be identified and discharge planning to be undertaken as early as possible in the patient's course of treatment.

The Department of Social Work Services, in response to the pressures for more rapid discharge planning, developed a pre-admission screening program. The social worker in the program was responsible for phoning each patient 65 years-of-age or older scheduled for elective admission in order to discuss the potential need for post-hospital planning and services. During the start-up phase of the project, only elective admissions were contacted; later, emergency room admissions were screened as well.

The social worker completed a psychosocial screening form for each patient contacted by phone or screened in the emergency room. This form included basic identifying information, diagnosis, and an assessment of psychosocial factors related to the need for post-hospital care, including assessment of various functional areas (ambulation, memory, etc.); an assessment of financial resources and entitlements; and an assessment of family supports and other resources available to the patient upon discharge (see Appendix). A combination of these factors resulted in the development of an overall rating to predict the likelihood that the patient will need post-hospital care. Three risk levels were identified: Risk Level 1–no need for services; Risk Level 2–potential need depending on medical outcome; and Risk Level 3–definite need for discharge planning services. Those cases coded Risk Level 3 have at least one further social work contact during the patient's stay.

During the first year of operation, 1414 patients were screened– 1058 elective patients, and 356 emergency room (ER) admissions. Of the electives, 241, or 23 percent, were assessed as being Risk Level 3, and of the ER admissions, 151, or 33 percent, were so coded. Thus, a significant proportion of the cases identified through the program were assessed as posing potential discharge problems.

Data gathered by the pre-admission screening social worker during a two-month period in 1987 were aggregated and analyzed.

A total of 234 cases were included in the analysis. Three sets of data analyses were generated: (1) descriptive data on the client population (2) examination of possible associations among psychosocial factors, and (3) examination of associations among various psychosocial factors and length of stay.

Aggregate descriptive findings were generated on age, living arrangements, income source, benefits, problem areas, and availability of natural support systems. Thirty-one percent of the clients in the study were between 65 and 69 years-of-age. Sixty percent of the clients in the study were 74 years or age or less. Fifty-seven percent of the population was female. Eighty-eight percent of the client population was receiving Social Security, and sixty percent was receiving a pension. The vast majority of the population resided in a house (a total of 81 percent). Very few of the clients were receiving any type of additional benefits such as food stamps, fuel assistance, or subsidized housing, and only six percent of the population were on Medicaid. Thus, the population reflected the relative affluence of the New York City metropolitan/suburban area in which the medical center is located.

Twenty-three percent of the clients in the study population reported living alone, while 54 percent lived with a spouse. With respect to support systems available to clients in the study population, 88 percent of the clients reported access to one or more helping persons. In most of these cases, the helper was the patient's spouse (52 percent), while in 19 percent of the cases an adult child was reported available to lend assistance. Thus, the population had access to social as well as material supports.

Finally, aggregate findings were generated regarding the functional problem areas identified by patients or their families at the time of the pre-admission screening. The two most common problem areas identified were difficulties walking (24 percent), and difficulties climbing stairs (24 percent). Problems with household tasks, shopping, and self-care skills such as bathing, dressing, and toileting were infrequently reported. Thus, the population was relatively well-functioning prior to their admission to the medical center.

A second set of data analyses was undertaken in order to determine whether there were any significant associations among age, living arrangements, and material supports. This involved the generation of a series of chi-square analyses among these variables. None of the findings were statistically significant.

In order to determine which psychosocial variables might be expected to affect length of stay, several analyses were conducted. It was hypothesized that individuals living with another household member might be expected to have lower overall lengths of stay than those who lived alone, because the availability of a key helper in the client's household generally facilitates discharge back to the home setting with home care supports in cases where the patient's medical condition does not require institutionalization. A t-test comparing average length of stay between those patients living alone and those living with another household member did not, however, produce a significant finding (p = .492).

A second analysis involved computation of an analysis of variance in order to determine whether age alone might have an impact on length of stay. The findings once again did not approach a level of statistical significance (F prob.–.8885). Finally, a stepwise regression analysis was computed in order to examine which functional deficiencies were most significantly associated with longer lengths of stay. The analysis examined the impact of the following problems: walking, climbing stairs, memory, dressing, bathing, toileting, completing chores, and shopping, and the additional variables of age, living alone, and DRG grouping (MDCS). Of the eleven variables included in the analysis, three were found to be significantly associated with length of stay: problems with memory, problems climbing stairs, and DRG diagnosis. This identifies indicators which can be useful to pre-admission screening workers in identifying high-risk cases (see Table 1).

A second important finding is that differences in mean length of stay were highly statistically significant among the three risk levels. The mean length of stay for patients who received a rating of Risk Level 1 was 5.9 days, for those receiving a rating of Risk Level 2, 9 days, and for patients receiving a rating of Risk Level 3, 12.9 days. An analysis of variance among these three groups was significant at the .05 level (see Table 2). This confirms that the psychosocial assessment protocol being utilized by the program, which includes an analysis of concrete, financial, and social resources available to

TABLE 1. Variables Significantly Associated with Length of Stay (memory, climbing stairs, and DRG diagnosis)

Variable	B	SE B	BETA	T	SIG T
MEMPROB	16.83812	4.80024	.22372	3.508	.0005
STRPROB	3.14326	1.25026	.15731	2.514	.0126
DRGDX	.26.57	.12761	.13019	2.042	.0423
(Constant)	5.95914	1.12522		5.296	.0000

TABLE 2. Risk Levels and Mean Length of Stays

	X LOS
Risk Level I	5.907
Risk Level II	9.000
Risk Level III	12.878
ANOVA	statistically significant

p = .05

patients, in conjunction with functional disabilities and medical condition, is effective in identifying high-risk cases which might be expected to pose discharge difficulties.

Another important finding is that cases admitted through the emergency room had an average length of stay that was significantly higher than cases admitted for elective procedures. (Analyses of referral source were based on a larger sample of 606 patients representing a two-month period in 1986 and the same two-month period in 1987.) As shown in Table 3, the mean length of stay for emergency room admissions was 11.6 days, while the average LOS for general elective admissions was 7.7 days; t-test analysis reveals a difference significant at the .05 level. This finding is consistent with the research of Munoz et al. (Munoz et al., 1986; Munoz et al., 1985; Munoz et al., 1986a; Munoz et al., 1986b), which revealed that emergency room admissions had higher overall costs than other cases regardless of the DRG diagnosis. This finding has important

TABLE 3. Length of Stay: Emergency Room and Elective Admissions

	X LOS
ER	11.5882
Elective	7.6716
Admissions	

t = − 5.24   p = .05

statistically significant

implications for social work departments wishing to contribute to more efficient discharge planning and more timely hospital releases. At LIJ, partially as a result of these findings, evening and weekend ER social work staffing was established.

A final significant finding was that the mean age for patients coming into the system through the emergency room was significantly higher than that for patients entering through regular elective channels. The mean age for emergency room patients was 76.7, while that of general admission patients 72.7; (p = .031). To the extent that greater age is independently associated with higher lengths of stay, this might help to explain the longer length of stay for emergency room patients (see Table 4).

DISCUSSION

The study of the pre-admission screening program identified selected psychosocial factors which may be identified as valid predictors of longer lengths of stay. Predictors or indicators may differ by institution or population (Coulton, 1988a). The identification of high-risk cases extends the period of time that social workers have to develop appropriate discharge plans for patients. Given the current cost-containment climate, social workers may be expected to face increasing pressure to discharge patients rapidly. A pre-admission screening program can facilitate the identification of high-risk cases earlier in the discharge planning process as well as the orchestration of appropriate post-hospital resources. Thus, timely discharges can be effected without compromising high quality patient

TABLE 4. Age, Emergency Room and Elective Admissions

	X AGE
ER	76.6912
ELECTIVE	76.6652
ADMISSIONS	

t = −6.37   p = .031

Statistically Significant

care. This is especially critical given recent demographic trends concerning health care utilization by the elderly, as well as trends concerning community resources. (New York's population over the age of 65 is the second largest in the nation, growing 7.4 percent between 1980 and 1985.) The elderly represent over 13.1 percent of the total population, or about 1 in 8 New Yorkers.* The number of people age 65 and older on Long Island has nearly doubled since 1960 and totalled more than 250,000 in 1980. More than 100,000 people were 75 or older in 1980.** For Nassau County alone, 12.4 percent of the population was 65 years-of-age or older in 1985, and it is projected that in 1990, 14 percent of the population will fall into the elderly category (Nassau County Planning Commission, *Nassau County, New York Data Book*, Mineola, New York, 1985). Nationally, by 1990, 12.6 percent of the U.S. population will be 65 and over; and 5.4 percent will be 75 and over (National Association of Social Workers, 1987). Reflecting these statistics, at LIJ, 12.9 percent of the total patient population in 1988 were 75 years-of-age or older, 25.9 percent of total inpatient days were utilized by patients 75 years-of-age or older. Based on a 4.2 percent annual increase, which is consistent with demographics for this area, by 1995, 22 percent of all patients at LIJ will be over the age of 75, utilizing 55 percent of inpatient days.

Reports from the National Center for Health Statistics (1985) affirm that chronic incapacities requiring dependency on others for assistance in mobility and personal care increase with age. Thus, the

---

*New York State Office of Aging.
**Nassau County Department of Senior Citizen Affairs.

need for supervised care can be expected to increase at the same time that community resources geared toward serving a dependent elderly population remain inadequate. There have been cutbacks in all continuing care services in the community, as well as cutbacks in Medicare home care services. In addition, there remain shortages of home attendants, home health aides, and nursing home beds. Pre-admission screening programs take on increased importance in light of these trends, to the extent that they allow workers greater time to plan for and execute discharge plans for the elderly.

A second purpose that can be served by pre-admission screening programs is the promotion of cost savings for hospitals as they attempt to maintain fiscal integrity under PPS. Under the PPS/DRG system, as opposed to the former cost-based system, every decrease in length of stay is translated into an immediate financial benefit for the institution. The field of hospital social work must take full advantage of the opportunity inherent in the present environment in order to gain a strong foothold in an area that is both financially critical to the survival of hospitals and crucial to the maintenance of quality of care for patients (Coulton, 1988b).

Finally, it should be noted that the prospective payment system methodology is designed to predict inpatient hospital resource utilization. The system sets standards based on medical diagnosis (diagnostic related groups–DRGs), but it ignores psychosocial characteristics which often determine discharge options and therefore, directly affect a patient's length of stay. The DRG methodology should be modified to incorporate psychosocial factors.

CONCLUSION

Pre-admission screening programs are a viable programmatic option to assist in timely and appropriate discharge planning, to minimize protracted lengths of stay resulting from difficulties in orchestrating discharge options, and to enhance the role of social work from both an organizational and from a service point of view. More research of the kind described in this article must be developed in this critical area affecting patient well-being and perhaps the survival of hospitals in an age of health care rationing.

APPENDIX. Pre-Admission Assessment Form

Department of Social Work Services
Long Island Jewish Medical Center

YOUR NAME: _____
ADDRESS: _____

DATE OF BIRTH: _____
DATE OF ADMISSION: _____

LIVING ARRANGEMENTS: _____

IF YOU HAVE STAIRS, HOW MANY STEPS? _____
Unknown _____

( ) house
( ) furnished room
( ) apartment
( ) adult home
( ) senior citizen housing
( ) skilled nursing facility
( ) health related facility
( ) other _____

(check as many as apply)
SOURCE OF INCOME:

( ) social security
( ) pension
( ) veteran's benefits
( ) social security disability
( ) public assistance
( ) other (specify) _____

WHO DO YOU LIVE WITH:

( ) alone
( ) husband/wife
( ) child
( ) other relative
( ) friend
( ) other

BENEFITS:

( ) subsidized housing
( ) Medicaid
( ) food stamps
( ) fuel assistance
( ) other (specify) _____

( ) uncertain

HOW LONG HAVE YOU HAD THESE
LIVING ARRANGEMENTS? _____

APPENDIX (continued)

DO YOU HAVE PROBLEMS WITH: (check as many as apply)

( ) walking   ( ) climbing stairs   ( ) dressing   ( ) bathing
( ) toileting   ( ) forgetfulness   ( ) housecleaning   ( ) shopping

DURING THE PAST SIX MONTHS, HAVE YOU HAD HELP WITH ANY OF THE FOLLOWING?

( ) household chores   ( ) bathing   ( ) dressing   ( ) cooking

IS THERE SOMEONE WHO WOULD BE ABLE TO HELP YOU AT HOME AFTER DISCHARGE FROM THE HOSPITAL?
( ) yes   ( ) no

( ) husband/wife   Helper's name: _____
( ) child   Home telephone: _____
( ) other relative   Business telephone: _____
( ) friend/neighbor   Best time to call: _____
( ) other
( ) uncertain

REFERENCES

Aaron, H. J., & Schwartz, W. B. (1984). *The painful prescription: Rationing hospital care.* Washington, DC: The Brookings Institution.

Berkman, B., & Rehr, H. (1970). Unanticipated consequences of the case-finding system in hospital social service. *Social Work, 15,* 63-68.

Berkman, B., & Rehr, H. (1972). The sick-role cycle and the timing of social work intervention. *Social Service Review, 46,* 567-580.

Berkman, B., & Rehr, H. (1973). Early social service case finding for hospitalized patients: An experiment. *Social Service Review, 47,* 256-265.

Berkman, B., Rehr, H., & Rosenberg, G. (1980). A social work department develops and tests a screening mechanism to identify high-risk situations. *Social Work in Health Care, 5*(4), 373-375.

Berkman, B., Bedell, D., Parker, E., McCarthy, L., & Rosenbaum, C. (1988). Preadmission screening: An efficacy study. *Social Work in Health Care, 13*(3), 35-50.

Boone, C. R., Coulton, C. J., & Keller, S. M. (1981). The impact of early and comprehensive social work services on length of stay. *Social Work in Health Care, 7*(1), 1-9.

Caputi, M. A., & Heiss, W. A. (1984). The DRG revolution. *Health and Social Work, 9*(1), 5-12.

Coulton, C. J. (1988a). Evaluating screening and early intervention: A puzzle with many pieces. *Social Work in Health Care, 13*(3), 65-72.

Coulton, C. J. (1988b). Prospective payment requires increased attention to quality of post hospital care. *Social Work in Health Care, 13*(4), 19-30.

Coulton, C. J., Dunkle, R. E., Goode, R. A., & MacKintosh, J. (1982). Discharge planning and decision making. *Health and Social Work, 7*(4), 253-261.

Glass, R. I., & Weiner, M. S. (1976). Seeking a social disposition for the medical patient: CAAST, a simple and objective clinical index. *Medical Care, 14*(7), 641-737.

Herman, J. M., Culpepper, L., & Franks, P. (1984). Patterns of utilization, disposition, and length of stay among stroke patients in a community hospital setting. *Journal of the American Geriatrics Society, 32*(6), 421-426.

Munoz, E., Soldano, R., Laughlin, A., Margolis, I. B., & Wise, L. (1986a). Source of admission and cost: Public hospitals face financial risk. *American Journal of Public Health, 76*(6), 696-697.

Munoz, E., Byun, H., Patel, P., Laughlin, A., Margolis, I. B., Wise, L. (1986). Surgonomics: The cost dynamics of craniotomy. *Neurosurgery, 18*(3), 321-326.

Munoz, E., Laughlin, A., Regan, D. M., Teicher, I., Margolis, E. B., & Wise, L. (1985). The financial effects of emergency department-generated admissions under prospective payment systems. *Journal of the American Medical Association, 254*(13), 1763-1771.

Munoz, E., Soldano, R., Sherrow, K., Laughlin, A., Margolis, I. B., & Wise, L.

(1986b). Mode of admission and cost for surgical DRGs. *Annals of Emergency Medicine, 15*(11), 21-27.

Nassau County Planning Commission. (1985). *Nassau County New York Data Book.* Mineola, New York.

National Association of Social Workers. (1987). *Face of the nation 1987: Statistical supplement to the 18th edition of the encyclopedia of social work* (National Association of Social Workers). Silver Spring, MD.

National Center for Health Statistics. (1985). *Health, United States, 1985* [Department of Health and Human Services (HHS)]. Hyattsville, MD.

Patchner, M. A., & Wattenberg, S. H. (1985). Impact of diagnosis related groups on hospital social service departments. *Social Work, 30*(3), 259-261.

Reamer, F. G. (1985). Facing up to the challenge of DRGs. *Health and Social Work, 10*(2), 85-94.

Reardon, G. T., Blumenfield, S., Weissman, A. J., & Rosenberg, G. (1988). Findings and implications from preadmission screening of elderly patients waiting for elective surgery. *Social Work in Health Care, 13*(3), 61-63.

Rock, B. D. (1987). Beyond discharge planning. *Hospital and Community Psychiatry, 38,* 529.

Rossen, S., & Colton, C. (1985). Research agenda for discharge planning. *Social Work in Health Care, 10*(4), 55-61.

Schrager, J., Halman, M., Myers, D., Nichols, R., & Rosenblum, L. (1978). Impediments to the course and effectiveness of discharge planning. *Social Work in Health Care, 4,* 65-80.

Vielhaber, D., & Irwin, N. (1975). Accounting for social work services in discharge planning (preliminary results of a survey). In *Quality Assurance in Social Services in Health Programs for Mothers and Children,* edited by W. T. Hall & G. C. St. Denis. (pp. 94-102). Pittsburgh: University of Pittsburgh Press.

Wolock, I., & Schlesinger, E. G. (1986). Social work screening in New Jersey hospitals: Progress, problems and implications. *Health and Social Work, 11*(1), 15-24.

POPULATION ISSUES

Significant changes in population distribution and need in this country have influenced personalities, values, and institutions that bring about a market change in the functioning of society as a whole. These changes have been most dramatic within the institution of the family where they have had a most telling effect on personal lives. Poverty, as an independent factor, is arguably the single most important determinant of health status in the United States. Low birth weight, malnutrition, and housing are a few examples of how poverty can impact health care and utilization rates. This section will examine teen pregnancy through the eyes of young fathers, health care strategies for Asian Americans, and changing roles in families.

Chapter 9

Adolescent Fathers: An Approach for Intervention

Neela P. Joshi
Stanley F. Battle

SUMMARY. Many myths exist concerning the needs and problems confronting adolescent fathers. Research on adolescent pregnancy has proliferated in the last decade. We now have a substantial body of empirically based findings in this area. Unfortunately, few substantive findings are available on adolescent fathers, yet the magnitude of this problem has reached epidemic proportion.

This chapter will provide an overview of current research on adolescent fathers and their needs and offer suggestions for appropriate intervention.

One important change affecting the U.S. family is an increasing delay in marriage and childbearing; but paradoxically, an increase in the number of adolescent parents. Until recently, adolescent parenthood was largely considered a woman's issue with the adolescent father being viewed as a "shadowy unknown figure, more a culprit than a potential contributor to either the mother or his offspring."[1] Traditionally, the adolescent father has received scant attention from social scientists, the judicial system, health care professionals, and policy makers.

Services and research in areas of sexual behavior, pregnancy, and parenting have usually concentrated on adolescent females. Nonetheless, there is evidence that successful pregnancy prevention pro-

This chapter was originally published in *Journal of Health & Social Policy*, Vol. 1(3) 1990.

grams for adolescents need to include males.[2] A recent survey regarding service programs for pregnant teenagers showed that a majority of U.S. cities have special programs for teenagers, but only a fourth provide services to male partners.[3] In a 1980 review, Earls and Siegel pointed out the paucity of research regarding teenage fatherhood;[4] however since then, some gains have been achieved.[5]

ADOLESCENT PREGNANCY: DEMOGRAPHIC FACTORS

In 1985 there were 477,705 infants–12.7% of all U.S. births–born to women 19 years of age and under.[6] According to the 1983 Urban League report, there are an estimated 1.3 million children living with 1.1 million adolescent mothers.[7] Prevalence of teenage fatherhood is also high. For example, in 1985, 107,650 births–22% of all births to teenage mothers–were to males 19 years of age and under.[8] It is believed that this figure represents considerable under-reporting. Many teenage mothers are unmarried and do not provide information regarding the father on the infant's birth certificate which is the source of prevalence data. The risk of becoming an adolescent father is high for black males due to a high prevalence of sexual activity and a low use of contraception.[9] The number of births/1000 unmarried, 15-19 years old, was more than six times greater among nonwhite than white.[10] Significant numbers of mothers, brothers, and sisters of teen fathers were teen parents themselves.[11]

Typically, the adolescent father and his partner are about the same age.[12] In a New Haven study of pregnant girls ≤ 17-years old, the average age of the father was 18.5 years, with 66% between 17 and 19 years old.[13] In Hendricks' study, 50% of the males were ≤ 17 years of age when they became fathers; and in a descriptive study of 26 fathers from Charlotte, N.C., the father's mean age was 18.7 years.[14] In most studies and reviews a majority of the adolescent fathers are described as unmarried at the time they become fathers and most come from low-income families.

In general, teenage fathers tend to be concentrated in the lower-paying, less prestigious occupations. They fare significantly worse probably because they obtain substantially less education and have lower income levels compared to adolescent males who postpone parenting until adulthood.[15] A majority of the teenage fathers work only part-time–usually at low wages–or are unemployed. Unemployment among black adolescent males in urban areas is approximately 37.3%.[16] In the New Haven study, the basic information on the fathers was obtained from 180 pregnant girls.[17] Fifty percent of these fathers were employed; 40% were enrolled in school with nearly 50% of those in school also working; and less than 5% were out of school and unemployed. In Hendricks' study of 21 black adolescent fathers (with 21 controls) fathers were less likely to be attending any type of school and more likely to be employed.[18]

Due to the cross-sectional nature of some of these studies,[19] obtaining information on the adolescent father only once regarding school or employment may lead to an erroneous impression. Given appropriate help and support, adolescent fathers are anxious to find jobs and finish their education according to the Bank Street College Project. The project funded by the Ford Foundation and coordinated by the Bank Street College of Education in New York–offered vocational services, counseling, and prenatal and parenting classes to approximately 400 teenage fathers and prospective fathers in eight U.S. cities. At the end of the two-year program, 61% of the previously unemployed adolescent fathers had found jobs and 46% of those who had dropped out of school had resumed their education.[20]

ADOLESCENT FATHERS: SEXUALITY AND CONTRACEPTION

Premarital sex among adolescents has been relatively common and generally acceptable for men.[21] A 1979 national survey of adolescent sexuality in the U.S. found that 70% of young men under age 21 had initiated intercourse before the age of 18 years.[22] The mean age of the first experience of sexual intercourse for a sample of 421 males from New York City high schools was: 11.6 years for blacks, 13 years for Hispanics, and 14.5 years for whites. Of the sexually experienced males, 97% had had their first experience before the age of 17.[23]

The use of contraceptives by adolescent males appears to be low. In a survey of three New York City high schools, 69% of the total sample of 421 reported that they were sexually experienced. Of those sexually experienced, 55% of the white males, 22% of the black males, and 19% of the Hispanic males reported using a contraceptive at last intercourse.[24]

The low mean age of first sexual experience and infrequent use of contraceptives in black males may be due to a different set of normative expectations regarding general heterosexual behaviors than their white counterparts. Advanced levels of heterosexual interaction among black preadolescent boys have been reported by Broderick.[25] Westney et al. assessed sexual maturation and sociosexual behaviors in a sample of 101 nine- to 11-year-old middle- and low-income boys and girls. The assessment regarding heterosexual behaviors was classified on a five-point heterosexual physical activity scale: game playing; holding hands, hugging or kissing; light petting; heavy petting; and intercourse. The researchers concluded that the sexual behaviors of preadolescent black males were heavily distributed in more advanced categories.[26] In a similar study of adolescents aged 12-15 years, black teens showed less precoital behavior and often had intercourse without any prior petting behaviors.[27] These behavior patterns may enhance the risks for unprotected intercourse and resultant unwanted pregnancy in young black adolescents.

In addition, for most young men intercourse is often a spur-of-the-moment decision.[28] Compared to female adolescents, males are less likely to recognize the risk of pregnancy; have less information about contraception; fewer formed attitudes that support contraceptive use; and greater reluctance to engage in what were perceived as female concerns.[29] In a sample of 421 males surveyed from three New York City high schools, 54% deemed birth control for girls only.[30] In a sample of 1,017 young male status offenders, 48% considered pregnancy to be the girl's fault because she should protect herself.[31] From these two studies, 70% and 61% respectively thought it was alright to have sex even if a couple was not in love.[32] Thus, sexual activity is viewed by male adolescents as casual and part of normal adolescent behavior.

Studies noted earlier regarding contraception in teen males do not reveal fatherhood status.[33] When these studies are compared with studies of adolescent fathers for variables such as age at first intercourse and mean age of intercourse, no differences are observed. However, in comparison to the studies on teen males where fatherhood status is unknown, studies on adolescent fathers show interesting differences regarding attitudes towards sex, their female partners, and contraceptive use. For example, in a study of 26 fathers from Charlotte, North Carolina, only nine (35%) reported using contraceptives prior to their partner's pregnancy; ten (38%) did not; and seven (27%) chose not to respond.[34] In the same study, 50% did not even raise the possibility of pregnancy. In a study of 33 expectant, black, teen couples, Brown concluded that these couples intended to resume their sexual relations after the birth of their child, but few knew the most effective method of birth control.[35] In the same study, 91% of the black expectant fathers disagreed with the premise that most black young men think getting a girl pregnant is evidence of their manhood.[36] Approximately 79% of the 95 unmarried, black teen fathers in one study reported it was wrong to tell a girl they loved her in order to have sex.[37] Also, two studies reported approximately 81% of expectant, black, unmarried adolescent fathers did not agree that the pregnancy was their female partners' fault.[38] Yet only 57% in one study thought a man should use a method of birth control whenever possible.[39]

Attitudes toward contraceptive responsibility and feelings toward one's partner may change as adolescent males move from nonfather to father status. Longitudinal studies that observe cohorts of adolescent males who move to fatherhood status would be useful.

ADOLESCENT FATHERS: ATTITUDES TOWARD ABORTION

Abortion appears to be a frustrating and emotionally costly experience to an unmarried male.[40] Black adolescent males tend to think abortion is wrong.[41] In a questionnaire administered to 41 black male partners of unmarried, adolescent pregnant and/or parenting females, only three (7.3%) would have chosen abortion; 28 (68.3%) wanted their partner to continue the pregnancy and keep the baby; two (4.7%) would have wanted their partner to continue the pregnancy and give the baby up for adoption; and eight (19.5%) were unsure.[42] A study of 95 black, unwed, adolescent fathers revealed that 93% did not want their partner to have an abortion, and 83% stated it was wrong.[43]

PSYCHOLOGICAL CORRELATES
OF ADOLESCENT FATHERHOOD

Available information does not shed much light on the psychologic characteristics of adolescent fathers. Two cross-sectional studies did not find any difference in locus of control between adolescent fathers and nonfathers.[44] However, in a study of 48 black, unmarried adolescent fathers, it was found that in comparison to nonfathers, fathers were more likely to be externally oriented, irrespective of educational status.[45] Using multivariate discriminate function analysis, Williams-McCoy and Tyler concluded that adolescent fathers are likely to be less trusting than nonfathers.[46] A correlational analysis in the same study also suggested that those fathers who were less trusting had an external locus of control.[47]

Clinical depression, significant enough to require referral for counseling, has been reported in adolescent fathers.[48] Actually, one-third of male partners of predominately black, lower-class pregnant teenagers in two special maternity programs reported feeling depressed during their partners' pregnancies, with several reporting social isolation.[49] In one of these two studies[50] the males at risk for depression appeared to be less sure regarding the decision to continue the pregnancy; were less likely to maintain an ongoing relationship with their partner; and were more likely to perceive a negative attitude toward them from their partner's family. On the whole, it is difficult to interpret the findings on psychological variables from these studies due to small sample sizes,[51] lack of objective measures to ascertain depression,[52] cross-sectional designs[53] and measurements of depression while the subjects were in a crisis situation,[54] i.e., after becoming fathers.

THE ROLE OF THE ADOLESCENT FATHER:
COMMITMENTS AND CONCERNS

The adolescent father is important to the psychological development of both his partner and their child. Henderson describes several aspects of fathering including genetic input; helping to facilitate the practical world for the mother during the pre and postnatal period; at times being a mother surrogate; being a role model for children; assisting the separation-individuation process, the development of the superego, shaping and helping socialization; and helping cognitive and maturational development.[55] A father's involvement augments a mother's interest and affect toward the infant.[56] It has also been speculated that if fathers are given the opportunity to be involved with their infant in the early neonatal period, they participate more in caretaking in the post-hospital period.[57] This interaction is very important for adolescent fathers.[58]

An adolescent male who becomes a father is expected to embody the father role while he is still negotiating the developmental tasks of adolescence. Depending upon his own cognitive and psychosocial development, he may or may not be able to provide emotional support for a young mother and contribute to the nurturance of their offspring. In addition, several prejudicial social factors, including the economic and social-welfare systems,[59] exclude adolescent fathers from continuing the relationship with their partners and actively participating in their children's upbringing: often the adolescent father is unmarried and physically separated at the time of the child's birth and early childhood, thereby reducing the number of opportunities available for interaction with the infant. Reportedly, 50% of adolescent fathers abandon their partners after pregnancy.[60] A teen father's absence leads to a common misconception of noncaring among health care providers who often perceive adolescent fathers as irresponsible deserters of their children. The divorce rate for adolescent parents is five times higher than for adults.[61] Also, the unrealistic expectations of adolescent mothers about the father's marriage plans coupled with the reality that most adolescent fathers do not wish marriage, may further contribute to the negative view of the adolescent father so prevalent in the literature.

There are no large scale systematic investigations about the parental behaviors of adolescent fathers. However, from interviews conducted with teenage couples, adolescent fathers seem eager to discuss their roles, situations, troubles, feelings, and expectations about fatherhood,[62] but often end up talking about their lives as teenagers.[63] In a study of 47 black, unmarried adolescent fathers, the subjects reported positive feelings about fatherhood, and perceived loving relationships with the young expectant mother.[64] A fairly large study of 100 adolescent fathers with a comparison group of 100 adolescent nonfathers found that as a group, teenage fathers did not perceive the consequences of adolescent childbearing as particularly detrimental.[65] Yet another study reported that 84% of fathers (n = 26) felt obligated to meet certain responsibilities for the mother and baby and most showed high motivation in participating in the parenting experience, such as naming the child, providing financial support, or both.[66]

In Nettleton and Cline's study of 138 unmarried, adolescent mothers, 85% reported regular contact with the infant's father at the first prenatal interview; 50% were dating the father of their child two years postpartum; and 20% eventually married the father.[67] Essentially, similar findings are reported by Rivara et al.[68] In a five-year, follow-up study of 404 first-time pregnant adolescents, Furstenberg found that 21% of the fathers were still residing with their children five years after the birth, 20% visited their children at least once a week, and 20% visited their children irregularly.[69] There also appears to be an association between the naming patterns of the children, frequency of paternal contact, and child support.[70] Where parents were not married, but the father visited his offspring at least once a week, 48% of the male children were given their father's forename, middlename, or both. In comparison only 14% bore his name when the father was not in contact with the offspring. Children named after the father and having regular contact were more likely to receive financial support.[71]

In the Bank Street College Project, at the end of a two-year observation of approximately 400 teenage fathers, 82% had daily contact with their children, and 74% contributed to their child's financial support.[72] In a longitudinal study of 180 teenage mothers, 46% were married or dating the father of their baby 26 months after delivery, and 64% received financial support for the infant both at three and 15 months postpartum.[73] A descriptive study of 26 teen fathers showed that approximately 67% reported maintaining regular contact with the mother of their child.[74] Although the length of time this contact was maintained is not specified, the percentage maintaining contact compares favorably with Furstenberg's study.[75]

In a cross-sectional study of 41 unwed, adolescent, pregnant and/or parenting females–ranging between 20 weeks gestation to three months postpartum–all reported knowing who their baby's father was and 96% had informed their male partners about the pregnancy.[76] In an analysis of the 41 responses from the male partners in this study, 80.5% still dated the female, 75.6% helped her by giving her money, and 83.5% helped her "in some other way." These studies lead us to conclude that many adolescent fathers wish to maintain contact with their families and want to participate in the parenting experience but are unable to do so due to age, income, educational attainment and several prejudicial social factors including economic and social welfare systems.

ADOLESCENT FATHERS AND COMPETENCY IN PARENTING

Parental role differentiation begins in early infancy.[77] A mother usually spends more time in caretaking activities such as feeding and changing the infant than the father does. However, this does not translate into less competence on the part of the father. One possible way to measure competency is to determine the parent's sensitivity to the infant's cues, for example, in feeding.[78] Fathers have been observed to adjust their behavior appropriately in response to an infant's distress signals.[79] Observation studies of adolescent fathers in caretaking situations, however, have not thus far been reported.

Adolescent fathers often have poor knowledge of child health maintenance and developmental milestones.[80] They also tend to have inappropriate expectations about the development of their children. In one study, adolescent fathers expected such developmental milestones as social smiling, sitting alone, pulling up to standing, taking the first step and speaking a word to be reached much earlier than the age appropriate for these norms.[81] Meaningful conclusions from the study, however, are limited by the absence of any statistical analyses, lack of a non-adolescent comparison group, and the selection of a convenience sample of rural working-class couples.

ADOLESCENT FATHERS AND INFANT DEVELOPMENT

Preliminary evidence suggests that involvement of adolescent fathers with their children facilitates the child's cognitive and social development in preschool years. The cognitive performance of preschool children was positively related to the continuity of contact between the child and his adolescent father.[82] When social adjustment of preschool children, where both adolescent parents were involved, was compared with children of single mothers, the latter scored lower on self-esteem and trust.[83] Furthermore, in father-absent families, 43% of the children had two or more behavior problems including temper tantrums, dishonesty, and bedwetting compared to less than 33% of the children living with both parents.[84]

PROBLEMS AND NEEDS OF ADOLESCENT FATHERS

Service programs that have worked with adolescent fathers report that adolescent fathers have multiple anxieties, stressors, and concerns.[85] The stressors for an adolescent father include worries about providing financial support to his new family; maintaining or getting a job; possibly not being able to finish school; events occurring during labor and delivery; and what the welfare and health of the child will be.[86] Teen fathers have an underlying fear of marriage and of responsibilities of fatherhood. They have difficulty in coping with the pregnancy and often have a need for counseling services. They also need information regarding reproductive physiology, childbirth, and children.[87] These anxieties and needs change in intensity over time. For example, in the Elster and Panzarine study, concerns about labor, delivery, and the mother's and infant's health were found from middle to the end of pregnancy, due probably to the inherent nature of this group of concerns.[88] Other concerns such as getting a job or finishing school, remained throughout the study.

A study that assessed the emotional needs of adolescent fathers reported significantly more difficulty in coping with the pregnancy and a more negative initial reaction in a group of adolescent fathers who showed lower adjustment on the Offer Scale of Self-Esteem.[89]

In many studies, adolescent fathers were found to have a substantial need for health education about reproductive physiology, childbirth and childcare, child development; information about employment; and counseling about coping with family life.[90] In a study of 33 expectant, black adolescent couples, the two most frequently cited concerns by teen fathers were future financial responsibility and their difficulty in finding a job.[91] Most expectant fathers in this study did not anticipate parenting problems, probably due to a lack of knowledge about what is involved in having a child.

In a study of 95 black unwed fathers, 55% noted their major problems were restriction of freedom due to the child's arrival, responsibility of providing for the child, limited opportunities to see the child, and not getting along with the mother of the child and other members of her family.[92] Twenty-three percent reported their problems related to a lack of money or employment, and an inability to finish school. Only 10% said they were having a problem coping with being a father.[93] In the same study, 88% reported they would turn to their family, especially their mothers, for help with a problem.[94] Friends and community resources, such as social service agencies, were cited as likely sources for seeking help by only 11% and 1% of the population respectively.[95] A study of a small convenience sample of 20 adolescent fathers found that the expectant fathers used problem-focused, direct action to prepare for their parenting role and to cope with the stress created by their situation.[96] These strategies included assuming the role of a provider, helping the partner to prepare for the baby, and talking with other young fathers, married friends, and parents. Family members and friends, although sympathetic and supportive of the young father, are unlikely to be capable of addressing all his adjustment problems and emotional needs.

Unmarried fathers, including adolescents, also have to face the negative attitudes of many social agencies. There is a lack of conviction that adolescent fathers have an important role, and providers fail to encourage adolescent fathers to actively participate.[97] The 1972 Supreme Court decision *Stanley v. Illinois* established equal protection of the law for unmarried, natural fathers.[98] In *Rothstein v. Lutheran Social Services*, the Supreme Court overturned a Wisconsin court decision which held that a putative father has no pa-

rental rights and no right to notice of any hearing, prior to a pro-
ceeding in which the mother has consented to the adoption of her
child.[99] Also, according to the amended 1973 Texas Family Code,
the fact that an unmarried parent is a minor does not affect his/her
rights in adoption or paternity cases.[100] Although these legal decisions have forced agencies counseling unmarried mothers to consider the rights of fathers and involve them in services, fathers are
still viewed as perpetrators and mothers as victims. Many times the
adolescent father is asked to meet financial commitments but not
permitted the opportunity to help nurture his family. Service providers need to make the effort to understand the desires and barriers
faced by adolescent fathers and plan more aggressive strategies to
involve them in existing programs for teen mothers and their children.

NEEDS FOR RESEARCH AND SERVICES

Important progress has been made in recent years in understanding the adolescent male's sexuality, contraceptive behavior,
and problems and needs after becoming a father. However, scientific utility of many of these studies on teen fathers is limited due to
(1) collection of data on small, biased samples that are recruited
through pregnant and/or parenting females; (2) cross-sectional observations regarding social and psychological characteristics of teen
males while they are in a crisis situation, i.e., after they become
fathers; and (3) the lack of utilization of standardized measures for
social and behavioral characteristics of the populations under study.
Future research should focus on:

1. Longitudinal studies, with adequate sample sizes, to assess
   adolescent males' psychosocial and personality characteristics
   and if they are predictive of teen fatherhood.
2. Studies of sexual attitudes, contraceptive knowledge, and behavior of adolescent males;
3. Studies of adolescent couples–their commitment and decision-
   making processes about contraception;
4. A study of gender differences about parenting responsibilities;
5. Exploration of the meaning of competent functioning for the
   adolescent male;

6. Studies of the role and influence of the parents of adolescent couples on the decision to continue or not continue a pregnancy;
7. Studies of the structural characteristics of the play between adolescent fathers and their infants as it facilitates infant development.

Male involvement in family planning and infant health maintenance and development should be encouraged. Since adolescent males are less likely to recognize the risk of pregnancy and have less information about the use of contraceptives,[101] information and services must be provided to both male and female adolescents. Although it is logical that parents should take this responsibility, many are unable or unwilling to meet this need. For adolescent males, the main sources of information about sexuality and contraception are often the media and their school experience. Hence the following changes in service delivery are suggested:

1. Schools should adopt a curriculum on family planning and sexuality, provide comprehensive health care services that include support for youngsters who wish to abstain from sexual activity, as well as provide contraceptives for those who need them. In dealing with minority males, health providers should be aware of the early age of first intercourse, the lack of precoital petting behaviors, and the lack of influence by male peers.

The development of school-based health clinics in many cities to deal with some of these issues is an encouraging trend. In one program, nearly 35% of the students using the clinic requested family planning counseling. However, of that total, only 6.9% were males.[102] There are now over 61 clinic sites in the U.S. and another 100 being developed.[103] Unfortunately, scant data are available from these clinics regarding male contraceptive use or change in knowledge, attitudes, and behaviors regarding contraception.

2. Existing service programs for pregnant and parenting teens should make efforts to include males in prenatal and parenting classes to inform them about fetal development, the birth pro-

cess, and child care. More males could be reached and successfully involved in these programs if prevocational and employment counseling were routinely provided.

3. Hospital maternity wards should provide opportunities for adolescent fathers to learn and practice basic caretaking skills, and to allow extended contact with the infant in the early postpartum period. School-age fathers should be given paternity leave and counseled about child development and childcare. This may be best achieved by providing training classes in infant development and caretaking by childcare facilities near or in schools.

SUMMARY

Many adolescent fathers are trapped by limited education, family instability, and judgmental behavior on the part of families, schools, or providers. Frequently, they are from minority groups and their future is relatively bleak.[104]

Strategies need to be developed to strengthen the role and position of minority men in their respective families, communities, and society. These strategies need to involve family members, peers, health care services, schools and organizations such as the Urban League, Planned Parenthood, and churches. Appropriate considerations must be given to teaching and modeling responsibility and sustaining group identity.

REFERENCE NOTES

1. Parke, R.D., Power, T.G., and Fisher, T. An adolescent father's impact on the mother and child. *J. Social Issues*, 1980;36 (1):88-106.

2. Edwards, L.E., Steinman, M.E., Arnold, K.A., and Hakanson, E.Y. Adolescent pregnancy prevention services in high school clinic. *Fam Plann Perspect*, 1980; 12:6-14.

3. Wallace, H.M., Weeks, J., and Medina, A. Services for pregnant teenagers in the large cities of the United States, 1970-1980. *JAMA*, 1982;248 (8):2270-2273.

4. Earls, F.L. and Siegel, B. Precocious fathers. *Am J Orthopsychiatry*, July 1980;50 (3):469-480.

5. Elster, A.B. and Panzarine, S. Unwed teenage fathers: Emotional and health educational needs. *J. Adol Health Care*, Dec. 1980;1 (2):116-120; Hendricks, L.E., Howard, C.S., and Caesar, P.P. Help seeking behavior among select populations of black unmarried adolescent fathers: Implications for human services agencies. *Am J. Public Health*, 1981; 71:733-735; Hendricks, L.E. Unmarried black adolescent father's attitudes toward abortion, contraception and sexuality: A preliminary report. *J. Adol Health Care*, March 1982; 2:199-203; Barret, R.L. and Robinson, B.E. A descriptive study of teenage expectant fathers. *Family Relations*, July 1982; 31:349-352; Robinson, B.E., Barret, R.L. and Skeen, P. Locus of control of unwed adolescent fathers versus adolescent nonfathers. *Perceptual and Motor Skills*, 1983; 56:397-398; Elster, A.B. and Panzarine, S. Teenage fathers: Stresses during gestation and early parenthood. *Clin Pediatrics*, Oct. 1983; 700-703; Vaz, R., Smolen, P., and Miller, C. Adolescent pregnancy: Involvement of the male partner. *J. Adol Health Care*, Dec. 1983; 4:246-250; Hendricks, L.E. and Montgomery T. A limited population of unmarried adolescent fathers: A preliminary report of their views on fatherhood and the relationship with the mothers of their children. *Adolescence*, Spring 1983;XVIII (69):201-210; Hendricks, L.E. and Fullilove, R.E. Locus of control and the use of contraception among unmarried black adolescent fathers and their controls: A preliminary report. *J. Youth Adolescence*, 1983;12 (3):225-233; Hendricks, L.E., Robinson-Brown, D.P. and Gary, L.E. Religiosity and unmarried black adolescent fatherhood. *Adolescence*, Summer 1984;XIX (74):417-424; Hendricks, L.E., Montgomery, T.A. and Fullilove, R.E. Educational achievement and locus of control among black adolescent fathers. *J. Negro Ed.*, 1984;53 (2):182-188; Brown, S.V. The commitment and concerns of black adolescent parents. *Social Work Research and Abstracts*, Winter 1983;19 (4):27-34; Rivara, F.P., Sweeney, P.J. and Henderson, B.F. A study of low socio-economic status black teenage fathers and their nonfather peers. *Pediatrics*, April 1985;74 (4):648-656; Rivara, F.P., Sweeney, P.J. and Henderson, B.F. Black teenage fathers: What happens when the child is born? *Pediatrics*, July 1986;78 (1):151-158.

6. National Center for Health Statistics. Monthly vital statistics report. Vol. 36, No. 4, Supplement, July 17, 1987.

7. National Urban League 1983 Annual Report, National Urban League, Inc.

8. Nat. Cent. Health Stats., Monthly Report.

9. Johnson, L.B. and Staples, R.E. Family planning and the young minority male: A pilot project. *The Family Coordinator*, Oct. 1979, 535-543.

10. National Center for Health Statistics. Monthly vital statistics report: Natality Statistics. *DHHS publication*, 1979, 27 (11) supplement.

11. Rivara, Sweeney, and Henderson, low socio-economic fathers.

12. Babikian, H.M. and Goldman, A. A. study in teenage pregnancy. *Am J. Psychiatry*, Dec. 1971;128 (6):111-116; Howard, M. Improving services for young fathers. *Sharing* Spring 1975.

13. Lorenzi, M.E., Klerman, L.B., and Jekel, J.F. School-age parents, how permanent a relationship? *Adolescence*, Spring 1977;45:13-22.

14. Hendricks, Unmarried black fathers; Robinson, Barret, and Skeen, Locus of control.

15. Card, J.J. and Wise, L.L. Teenage mothers and teenage fathers: The impact of early childbearing on the parents' personal and professional lives. *Fam. Plann Perspective*, July/August 1978;10 (4):199-205.

16. *The Boston Sunday Globe*, June 14, 1987, A4.

17. Lorenzi, Klerman, and Jekel, School-age parents.

18. Hendricks, Robinson-Brown, and Gary, Religiosity and fatherhood.

19. Barret and Robinson, Teenage expectant fathers.

20. The Bank Street College of Education and Ford Foundation Project. *Time*, December 9, 1985:p.90.

21. Kinsey, A.C., Promeroy, W.B. and Martin, C.E. *Sexual behavior in the human male*. Philadelphia: W.B. Saunders 1948.

22. Zelnick, M. and Shah, F.K. First intercourse among young Americans. *Fam Plann Perspective* March/April 1983;15 (2):64-70.

23. Finkel, M.L. and Finkel, D.J. Sexual and contraceptive knowledge, attitudes and behavior of male adolescents. *Fam Plan. Perspect.*, Nov/Dec. 1975;7 (6):256-260.

24. Ibid.

25. Broderick, C.B. Social heterosexual development among urban negroes and whites. *J. Marriage and Family*, 1965; 27:200-203.

26. Westney, O.E., Jenkins, R.R., Butts, J.D., and Williams I. Sexual development and behavior in black preadolescents. *Adolescence*, 1984 (Fall) XIX 75:557-567.

27. Smith, E.A., Udry, J.R. Coital and non-coital sexual behaviors of white and black adolescents. *AJPH*, Oct. 1985 75 (10):1200-1203.

28. Zelnick and Shah, First intercourse.

29. Freeman, E.W., Rickle, K., Huggins, G., Mudd, E.H., Garcia, C-R, and Dickens, H.O. Adolescent contraceptive use: Comparison of male and female attitudes and information. *Am J Publ Health*, August 1980;7 (8):790-797.

30. Babikian and Goldman, Teenage pregnancy.

31. Vadies, E. and Hale, D. Attitudes of adolescent males toward abortion, contraception and sexuality. *Social Work in Health Care*, Winter 1977;3 (2):1969-1974.

32. Babikian and Goldman, Teenage pregnancy; Freeman, E.W., Rickle, K., Huggins, G., Mudd, E.H., Garcia, C-R, and Dickens, H.O. Adolescent contraceptive use.

33. Finkel and Finkel, Sexual and contraceptive knowledge; Zelnick and Shah, First intercourse; Freeman, E.W., Rickle, K., Huggins, G., Mudd, E.H., Garcia, C-R, and Dickens, H.O. Adolescent contraceptive use; Vadies and Hale, Attitudes toward abortion.

34. Barret and Robinson, Teenage expectant fathers.

35. Brown, Commitment and concerns.

36. Ibid.

37. Hendricks, Unmarried black fathers.

38. Ibid; Brown, Commitment and concerns.

39. Hendricks, Unmarried black fathers.

40. Rothstein, A.A. Adolescent males fatherhood and abortion. *J Youth and Adolescence*, 1978;7 (2):203-214; Shostak, A.B. Abortion as fatherhood lost: Problems and reforms. *Family Coordinator*, 1979;28:569-574.

41. Vadies and Hale, Attitudes toward abortion.

42. Vaz, Smolen, and Miller, Adolescent pregnancy.

43. Hendricks, Unmarried black fathers.

44. Robinson, Barret, and Skeen, Locus of control; Hendricks, Montgomery, and Fullilove, Educational achievement.

45. Hendricks, Montgomery, and Fullilove, Educational achievement.

46. Williams-McCoy, J.E. and Tyler, F.B. Selected psychological characteristics of black unwed adolescent fathers. *J Adol Health Care*, Jan. 1985;6 (1):12-16.

47. Ibid.

48. Elster and Panzarine, Unwed teenage fathers; Vaz, Smolen, and Miller, Adolescent pregnancy.

49. Ibid.

50. Vaz, Smolen, and Miller, Adolescent pregnancy.

51. Elster and Panzarine, Unwed teenage fathers; Robinson, Barret, and Skeen, Locus of control; Vaz, Smolen, and Miller, Adolescent pregnancy; Hendricks, Montgomery, and Fullilove, Educational achievement.

52. See note 48.

53. See note 51.

54. See note 48.

55. Henderson, J. On fathering (the nature and functions of the father role), Part II: Conceptualization of fathering. *Can J. Psychiatry*, August 1980;25:413-431.

56. Sawin, D.B. and Parke, R.D. Adolescent fathers: Some implications from recent research on paternal roles. *Educational Horizons*, Fall 1976;55 (1):38-43.

57. Parke, R.D. and O'Leary, S.E. Father-mother-infant interaction in the newborn period: Some findings, some observations and some unresolved issues. In Riegel, K. and Meachon, J. (Eds). The developing individual in changing world, Social Environmental Issues Vol. III. The Hague Mouton, 1976.

58. Sawin and Parke, Adolescent fathers; Parke and O'Leary, Father-mother-infant interaction.

59. Stack C.B. *All our kin strategies for survival in a black community*. Harper and Row, 1974.

60. Brown-Robbins, M.M. and Lynn, D.B. The unwed fathers: Generation recidivism and attitudes about intercourse in California youth authority wards. *J. Sex Research*, Nov. 1973;9 (4):334-341.

61. Connolly, L. Boy fathers. *Human Behaviors*, Jan. 1978; 40-43.

62. Ibid; Caparulo, F.L. and London, K. Adolescent fathers: Adolescents first, fathers second. *Issues in Health Care of Women*, Jan-Feb 1981;3 (1):23-33.

63. Caparulo and London, Adolescent fathers.

64. Hendricks and Montgomery, Limited population.

65. Rivara, Sweeney, and Henderson, Low socio-economic fathers.

66. Barret and Robinson, Teenage expectant fathers.

67. Nettleton, C.A. and Cline, D.W. Dating patterns, sexual relationships and use of contraceptives of unwed mothers during a two-year period following delivery. *Adolescence*, 1975;37:45-57.

68. Rivara, Sweeney, and Henderson, Black teenage fathers.

69. Furstenberg, F.F. The social consequences of teenage parenthood. *Fam. Plann Perspect* 1976;8:148-164.

70. Furstenberg, F.F. and Talvitie, K. Children's names and paternal claims. *J Fam Issues*, March 1980;(1):31-57.

71. Ibid.

72. Bank Street College, *Time*.

73. Lorenzi, Klerman, and Jekel, School-age parents.

74. Barret and Robinson, Teenage expectant fathers.

75. Furstenberg, Social consequences.

76. Vaz, Smolen, and Miller, Adolescent pregnancy.

77. Kotelchuck, M. The infant's relationship to the father: Experimental evidence. In M.E. Lamb (Ed.) *The role of the father in child development*. New York: Wiley 1976.

78. Parke, Power, and Fisher, Adolescent father's impact.

79. Ibid.

80. Rivara, Sweeney, and Henderson, Black teenage fathers.

81. DeLissovoy, V. Child care by adolescent-parents. *Children Today*, 1973;4:22-25.

82. Furstenberg, F.F., Jr. Unplanned Parenthood. New York Free Press 1976.

83. Ibid.

84. Ibid.

85. Elster and Panzarine, Stresses during gestation.

86. Ibid.

87. Pannor, R. and Evans, B.W. The unmarried father revisited. *The Journal of School Health* 1975;XLV (5):286-291; Panzarine, S. and Elster, A.B. Prospective adolescent fathers: Stresses during pregnancy and implications for nursing interventions. *J. Psychosoc Nurs Ment Health Serv*, July 1982;20 (7):21-24; Hendricks, L.E., Howard, C.S. and Caesar, P.P. Black unwed adolescent fathers: A comparative study of their problems and help seeking behavior. *J. Nat. Med. Association*, 1981;73 (9):863-868.

88. Elster and Panzarine, Stresses during gestation.

89. Elster and Panzarine, Unwed teenage fathers.

90. Ibid; Hendricks, Howard and Caesar, Help seeking behavior.

91. Brown, Commitment and Concerns.

92. Hendricks, Unmarried Black fathers.

93. Hendricks, Howard and Caesar, Comparative Study of problems.

94. Ibid.

95. Ibid.

96. Elster and Panzarine, Stresses during gestation.

97. Pannor, R. The teenage unwed father. *Clin Obstet and Gynecol*, 1971; 14:466-472.

98. Pannor and Evans, Unmarried father revisited.

99. Ibid.

100. *Vernon's Texas Codes Annotated: Family code with annotations, tables and index.* St. Paul, MN: West Publishing Co., 1973:230-241.

101. Zelnick and Shah, First intercourse.

102. Edwards, L.E., Steinman, M.E., Arnold, K.A., and Hakanson, E.Y. Prevention services.

103. Lovick, S.R. and Wesson, W.F. School Based Clinics: Update. 1986. Spring Center for Population Options–Washington, DC.

104. Barret and Robinson, Teenage expectant fathers; Rivara, Sweeney, and Henderson, Low socio-economic fathers; Brown-Robbins and Lynn, Unwed fathers; Card and Wise, Impact of early childbearing.

Chapter 10

Health Care Strategies
for Asian American Patients

Michael M. O. Seipel

SUMMARY. The health status of Asian Americans is at risk because the existing health care delivery system is unable to provide ethnic-sensitive health care services. This condition is attributed to the changing policies and practices of the health care system of the past decades. Thus it is argued that health care providers must become more knowledgeable about the specific health needs of Asian Americans.

As a result of advancements in scientific knowledge, improved nutrition, and social conditions in general, Americans enjoy better health today than ever. Today, Americans live longer, are less at risk from infectious diseases, and receive better treatment for various health problems. However, the overall advances in health developments in the United States have not fully met the health needs of ethnic minorities (Bullough & Bullough, 1982; U.S. Department of Health, 1985). This paper discusses specific issues and policies that affect the health care needs of Asian Americans in the United States.

SCOPE OF THE PROBLEM

Health status disparities exist between American whites and non-whites. Though Asian Americans in the aggregate are healthier than

This chapter was originally published in *Journal of Health & Social Policy*, Vol. 1(1) 1989.

all other racial ethnic groups, they are not without problems. For instance, the Report of the Secretary's Task Force on Black and Minority Health (U.S. Department of Health, 1985) shows that even though the rate for excessive death for Asian Americans is lower than expected, the risk for health problems increases when new immigrants are taken into account. If the current trend of immigration continues, the relative health risk for Asian Americans will be substantial. Already, 58% of 3.7 million Asian Americans are foreign born, and immigration from Asia/Pacific Islands is projected to increase (U.S. Department of Health, 1985).

There are a number of reasons why the health of immigrants is at a greater risk than the overall health of Americans. Chief among these is that Asian Americans are reluctant to use mainstream health care systems. In a UCLA study (cited in Harwood, 1981), Chinese Americans in Los Angeles substantially underused hospital care. Exact data are not available for other Asian American groups, but among Asians there appears to be a general underuse of mainstream medical services (U.S. Department of Health, 1985; Hesler et al., 1975).

OBSTACLES FOR ASIAN AMERICAN HEALTH CARE

Since the turn of the century, health care delivery systems have gone through some fundamental and useful changes, but paradoxically, they have also became less able to accommodate health needs of ethnic minorities. Consequently, health care in certain instances is outstanding, yet less than adequate in other instances, especially in meeting the specific health needs of recent immigrants from Asia (Schultz, 1982; U.S. Department of Health, 1985). The following serious obstacles prevent better health services to Asian Americans: (1) changes in patient physician relationship; (2) changes in provision of health care from community/home to hospitals; (3) changes in health training strategies; (4) discrimination.

Changes in Patient-Physician Relationship

In earlier decades, many physicians maintained one-to-one relationships with their patients; a relationship that emphasized informal and individualized care over formal and institutionalized care. Physicians were usually available when they were needed. Many physicians lived in the same neighborhood as their patients, because their economic circumstances were similar to those of their patients. At times fees reflected patients' ability to pay.

However, when medicine became more "scientific" and efficient, emphasis on individualized health care practice diminished because it was thought to be inefficient. As a result of this development, health care practice moved away from a person-oriented treatment approach to a disease-oriented approach. Asian American preference for a personal style of interaction with physicians then came into conflict with the practice of efficiency and impersonality embodied in the current health care system. Not surprisingly, Asian Americans and other disadvantaged patients were pushed further out of an individualized health care system (Bullough & Bullough, 1982).

Change from Community/Home to Hospital-Based Care

To an increasing extent, health care has become institutionalized. What was once treated in the home, now is treated in hospitals. Several events contributed to this trend. First, by the twentieth century, medical technology advanced and medical procedure improved. This led to a concentration of patients and physicians in hospitals so that both parties could more fully benefit from life-saving machines and techniques, as well as obtain a return on expensive medical investments. Second, the health care reimbursement system encouraged hospital-centered care over office-based or home-based care. Health insurance industries, both private and public, favored reimbursements on services rendered in hospitals. Consequently, many medical procedures and treatments that could be handled in the office or home were transferred to hospitals (Bullough & Bullough, 1982).

Moving the health care base from office/home to hospitals has made mainstream health care service less accessible to Asian Americans. This outcome was predictable. When treatment orientations changed, health facilities changed, and that led a migration of health facilities from minority neighborhoods to middle-class neighborhoods and university campuses. Facilities became even less accessible to Asian American patients. Moreover, Asian Americans were reluctant to seek out health services from hospitals, because many viewed hospitals to be at best impersonal, and at worst, a place to die (Harwood 1981).

Changes in Health Care Training Strategies

To upgrade both health services and income of health providers, education was dramatically upgraded. For instance, the length of training in medical schools increased, more specialized training was offered, and the number of students admitted to the program was deliberately lowered. A similar change took place in nursing and other allied health disciplines.

These developments were not without cost. To no one's surprise, upgraded education efforts caused the cost of education to skyrocket beyond the reach of many ethnic minority students. In addition, the training curriculum began to emphasize health needs of middle- and upper-class populations, while benignly ignoring special health needs of the poor and minorities. As a result, there are only a few ethnic minority health care providers to meet special health care needs of such patients, while health care providers in general do not have the training necessary to provide ethnic-sensitive health care services to Asian American patients (Bullough & Bullough, 1982).

Discrimination

The fruits of discrimination are found in health disparities between whites and nonwhites. The Report of the U.S. Department of Health (1985) shows that minorities are less healthy and receive less appropriate care. More specifically, the report shows that minorities have less information on health care, they see physicians less frequently than whites, and more are without health insurance coverage, or have inadequate coverage.

Today, minorities are not denied health care on the basis of race or color. But even if there is no overt racism or discrimination, there still exists a double standard for treating minority patients. Minority patients are often relegated to second-rate care because health providers are either unaware of or ignore their specific needs.

SPECIAL ISSUES TO BE CONSIDERED

A common theme in these health care obstacles is that the present health care system and providers are inadequately prepared to deal with the special issues and needs of Asian American patients. An institutional commitment could largely solve this problem. However, central to any effort that aims to provide better health care are health care providers. Physicians, nurses, social workers, and other direct care providers are the primary source of problem solvers. They are the ones who must take an initial leadership responsibility to provide better health care by becoming more knowledgeable of minority health challenges. The key concerns in treating Asian Americans are these: (1) understanding the Asian American's concept of health and illness; (2) involving the family in the treatment; (3) understanding the system of interaction.

Understanding the Concept of Health and Illness

Understanding the theory of illness can lead to more appropriate treatment strategies. For example, in Asia, health problems are thought to be brought on by imbalance or disharmony in lifestyle. Imbalance occurs when the body experiences either an excess of one or a deficiency of another, such as too much work, too little rest, boredom, too much tension, too much eating, not eating enough. This idea is embodied in the concept of the "hot" and "cold" system found in "Yin-Yang" polarity. Yin-Yang states that all things in the universe consist of two energy forces; and if harmony and health in mind and body are to be maintained, the two energy forces must be in perfect balance (Campbell & Chang, 1973; Topley, 1970).

Appropriate health care strategies can be formulated if providers have more information about the patient. This point is illustrated in the following case (Kleinman, Eisenberg, & Good, 1978).

Chang, a 33-year-old Chinese man (Cantonese speaking) came to the medical clinic of a general hospital complaining of tiredness, dizziness, general weakness, pain in the upper back, a sensation of heaviness in the feet, weight loss, and insomnia of six-months' duration. He denied any emotional complaints. Past medical history was noncontributory. Medical work-up was unrevealing except that the patient seemed anxious and looked depressed. However, he refused to acknowledge either of these feelings. He initially refused referral for psychotherapy, stating that talk therapy would not help him. Reluctantly, he finally agreed to see a social worker for counseling and a psychiatrist for medication. Both clinicians defined the problem as a depressive reaction. In contrast, Chang and his family defined it as due to "wind" (fung) and "cold" (leung) diseases. He reported that his health problem began two years ago when he returned to Hong Kong to find a wife. He acquired the "wind" disorder after having overindulged in sexual relations with prostitutes, which resulted in loss of "huethei" (blood and vital breath), causing him to suffer from "cold" (leung) and "not enough blood." His symptoms worsened after his wife's second miscarriage.

After seeking advice from his family and friends, the patient first began treating himself with traditional Chinese herbs and diet therapy. This involved both the use of tonics to "increase blood" and hot food to correct his underlying state of humoral imbalance. When he failed to improve, they suggested that he return to Hong Kong to consult a traditional Chinese practitioner there.

While the patient was seen at the clinic, he continued to use Chinese herbs and to seek out consultation and advice from friends, neighbors, and recognized "experts" in the Chinese community who frequently told him that his problem could not be helped by Western medical care. He also received help from an acupuncturist. Mr. Chang never told his family or friends about receiving mental health services. He expressed gratitude, however, that the social worker listened to his view about his problem and that he explained ideas about depression. He remembered feeling bad about his care in the medical clinic where the doctor never explained anything to him. He was grateful that he was receiving medication in the psychiatric clinic.

The patient improved with complete remission. He thanked the worker and the psychiatrist for their help, but confided that (1) he remained confident that he was not suffering from a mental illness;

(2) talk therapy had not been of help; (3) medication perhaps was effective against "wind" disorders; and (4) because he had concurrently taken a number of traditional Chinese herbs, it was uncertain what had been effective, and perhaps the combination of traditional Chinese and Western drugs had been responsible for the cure. (Kleinman, 1978, p. 253)

Involve Family

The family is the most important support system available to Asian Americans. They are ever-present when a patient is admitted to the hospital, and the family plays an important role in the patient's treatment process. Care providers must understand the strength of family commitment to solve health problems. Having a deep sense of obligation to care for their own, they do not wish to pass the responsibility to strangers (Chang, 1981).

Health care providers must be aware of the structure and role of family and its support system. This knowledge can be an invaluable frame of reference in assessing and treating Asian American patients. Chang (1981) points out that because the Korean American family is patriarchal, providers would do well to consider feelings and opinions of the father when the treatment decision is made. This point is illustrated in the following incident by Chang:

> An 8-year-old boy, a second-generation Asian, was hospitalized on a pediatric unit of a large metropolitan hospital with a diagnosis of multiple fractures following a bicycle accident. The 35-year-old mother, a first-generation Asian, spent most of the day in the hospital, and the father came after work each evening to visit the child. A stream of other visitors were in and out of the room all day bringing various foods for the young patient. Members of the staff expressed a variety of concerns, ranging from "the boy is being disturbed too much," "he is old enough to accept the separation from his parents," to being afraid the food would clutter up the room too much.
>
> The staff made a special effort to talk with the parents, because they were at first incommunicative even though they spoke some English. It was discovered that this was the only

son and first grandson in the family. The mother had felt she was to blame for "not watching him carefully enough." Rather than further discuss her feelings, she wanted to be able to "live in" at the hospital to ensure that the son was well taken care of, and her husband encouraged her to stay at the hospital to pay full attention to the child's needs. (p. 261)

On the basis of knowledge of the prescribed role of traditional Korean family, the provider revised the care plan to the satisfaction of the child's father by making a special arrangement to let the mother sleep on a cot in the child's room.

Understanding the System of Interaction

Treatment strategies are enhanced when a mutual understanding takes place in health care relationships. Traditional Asian interaction seeks to establish harmony and avoid conflicts between a patient and a care giver. This interaction is characterized by restraint, reserve, and nonassertiveness. A confrontation leads to loss of face and possible termination of the treatment process. In typical care-giving relationships, Asian American patients respect physicians because they are perceived to be learned, benevolent, serious, and polite. On the other hand, they also expect physicians to treat them with respect and decorum, especially when a patient is older than a physician (Harwood, 1981).

The same respect and decorum given to male patients needs to be extended to female patients. If a woman patient is particularly sensitive about intimate care given by a male physician, he should do all he can to protect her modesty.

This point is illustrated in the following case of a Native American woman (the principle also applies to Asian American women) (Primeaux & Henderson, 1981).

The morning after Ms. Z's admission, the nurse wishes to give her a bath and comb her hair. Because modesty is important to a Navajo, she asked permission. Asking permission of any adult patient prior to beginning a bath is good common sense, but it is especially important to Navajos because disrobing in front of strangers discomforts them. After the bath the nurse helped Ms. Z comb her hair. Then she removed all hair from the brush and saved it in the bedside stand. The Navajo dispose of it appropriately later. (p. 247)

CONCLUSION

Despite unprecedented growth of medical knowledge and technology, current health care arrangements are causing health disparities between whites and nonwhites in the United States. A careful examination shows that current health care practice lacks the cultural sensitivity necessary to treat Asian American patients. It is therefore argued that health care providers should assume a greater responsibility to include cultural components in their practice with Asian American patients.

REFERENCES

Bullough, V. L. & Bullough, B. (1982). *Health care for other Americans.* New York: Appleton-Century-Crofts.

Campbell, T. & Chang, B. (1973). Health of the Chinese in America. *Nursing Outlook, 21*(4), 245-249.

Chang, B. (1981). Asian-American patient care. In *Transcultural health,* edited by G. Henderson & M. Primeaux (pp. 255-278). Menlo Park, CA: Addison-Wesley Publishing Co.

Harwood, A. (1981). *Ethnicity and medical care.* Cambridge: Harvard University Press.

Hesler, R. M., Nolan, M. E., Ogbur, B., & New, P.K.M. (1975). Intraethnic diversity: Health care of the Chinese Americans. *Human Organization, 34*(3), 253-262.

Kleinman, A., Eisenberg, L., & Good, B. (1978). Illness, culture, and care. *Annals of Internal Medicine, 88*(2), 251-258.

Primeaux, M. & Henderson, G. (1981). American Indian patient care. In *Transcultural Health,* edited by M. Primeaux & G. Henderson (pp. 239-254). Menlo Park, CA: Addison-Wesley Publishing Co.

Schultz, S. C. (1982). How Southeast-Asian refugees in California adapted to unfamiliar health care practice. *Health and Social Work, 7*(2), 148-156.

Topley, M. (1970). Chinese traditional ideas and the treatment of disease: Two examples from Hong Kong. *Man, 5*(3), 421-437.

U.S. Department of Health. (1985). *Report of the secretary's task force on blacks and minority health.* Washington, DC: U.S. Government Printing Office.

Chapter 11

Changing Family Roles

Stanley F. Battle

Since 1960, changes in the social and political arenas have deeply influenced families in America. Increases in adolescent pregnancy rates, changes in childrearing practices, alternative life style groups, and a marked growth of divorce rates have influenced us all to some degree. The emergence of a new liberal philosophy has further impacted the social fabric.

In many instances, the black family has continued to adjust, as well as mold a new character in terms of marital patterns while maintaining the unique status of a minority. We have witnessed the emergence of an upwardly mobile black middle class. Unfortunately, racial prejudice and segregation are still rampant; blacks are especially judged with higher standards in the employment arena, which has a significant impact on the black family (Staples, 1981).

This chapter focuses on critical considerations and changing patterns of black family life in order to examine specific characteristics of the black family in the context of the 1980s. The family is at a crucial point in its development, given the pressures of unemployment, single-parent families, and changes in male-female relationships. In fact, the future of black children may be at stake.

HISTORICAL CONSIDERATIONS

It is impossible to adequately describe the impact of Africa on blacks from a historical point of view because of the unlimited

This chapter was originally published in *Journal of Health & Social Policy*, Vol. 1(4) 1990.

variations in the population, although it does appear the bulk of the slave trade was from West Africa. Africa was characterized by various forms of political organization. There were organized kingdoms and isolated family states where both had the capacity to establish governments for solving the problems that every community encountered. The family state prevailed in areas where territory was divided among a number of families, and where there was no desire on the part of these families to merge their resources in order to form a stronger state. In such a situation, the chief was very powerful because his political strength was supplemented by virtue of being head of the family. Further, it was not uncommon for several states to band together to form a more powerful state (Franklin, 1970).

For years the texts of Frazier (1939) and Elkins (1968) were accepted as the definitive histories of black families. A challenge to earlier scholarship came in 1972 from Blassingame (1972), who detailed that in slave quarters, black families did exist as functioning institutions and as role models. Strong family ties were established in spite of frequent break-ups resulting from breeding and the slave trade.

The slave family experienced great difficulty in maintaining itself on a stable basis in a system where so little opportunity for expression was possible (Frazier, 1939). Seldom did the owner recognize the slave family as an institution worthy of respect. Courtship and normal relationships that were preliminary to marriage seldom existed. Only when an owner manifested some real interest in the religious and moral development of his slaves was there an effort to maintain a stable slave family.

Probably one of the most important studies, by Gutman (1976), helped put myths to rest about the black family. He examined plantation birth records and marriage applications, and concluded that the dual-parent household was dominant during slavery. He also found that from 1880 to 1925 the majority of blacks were from nuclear families. Gutman's work helped to provide supportive evidence that slavery did not destroy the black family, and it was his contention that the black family evolved from established family and kinship patterns. But this did not prevent challenges to the black family that emerged during the 1960s (Gutman, 1976).

BLACK FAMILY STRUCTURES

There are two types of family structures in America male-headed and female-headed families. The general assumption is that male-headed families are more stable than families headed by women. This posture is undergoing considerable scrutiny today. Furthermore, female-headed families are assumed to be more commonly accepted among blacks; this appears to be an invalid belief.

It is important to reconceptualize various family structures. Billingsley (1968) points out that there are three general categories of families: primary (nuclear), extended, and augmented families. Nuclear families are confined to husband and wife and their children, with no other members present. Extended families encompass other relatives or in-laws sharing the same household with nuclear family members, while augmented families include members that are not related to the nuclear family but who share the same living situation (Billingsley, 1968). Examining these structural variables in relation to black families, the following broad questions may be helpful to professionals working with black families:

1. *Is the black family nuclear?* Is family structure representative of the "typical" family: that is, father, mother, and children all living together? If so, it is critical to ascertain member roles within that context. For example, many black families are egalitarian in decision making, with both the mother and father sharing these responsibilities. In other families, decision making is divided, with the mother having dominance in many areas, e.g., childrearing, household budgeting, moral training, etc., and the father being more concerned with discipline, home repairs, and broad-based budgeting. Whatever the roles, it is likely the family will initially present itself as being more "traditional," as one means of presenting a viable front to escape being perceived as "deviant."

2. *Is the black family extended?* The black extended family takes on many forms: it may be a nuclear family with the addition of a direct blood relative such as a grandparent, or a nuclear family that also includes the young children of daughters who may or may not live in the home. In many cases, the grandmother may often be called "mama" by her grandchildren. There are other variations, but, importantly, it is necessary to informally ascertain how the particular

extended family system functions in terms of roles, responsibilities, finances, and emotional supports. If the black extended family system includes the grandmother, then it is prudent to hypothesize that she probably wields significant influence on the cohesiveness, pattern-maintenance, and moral activities of the family.

3. *Is the black family augmented?* The augmentation may consist of a friend from the hometown, a child, or a church acquaintance who is being informally fostered, or a host, or other type of relationship. Again it is important to assess roles, responsibilities, financial and emotional reciprocity.

In many instances, little affectional distinction exists between augmented and blood relatives. A fairly common example of this is reflected by the black cultural style of informal adopting or fostering.

Historically, blacks have displayed a unity and tribal cohesiveness in which respect and trust were placed in other blacks to help provide direction and discipline for the children. It was understood that black people were responsible for black children and often, the protection took the form of harsh words or maybe even a slap to prevent a worse fate at the hands of "the man" (the white power structure). Physical discipline was accepted in black schools and, in most instances, a child knew that a spanking at school would be followed by a spanking for the misbehavior at home. Childrearing in the black community was not necessarily perceived as the task of parents. Often when a child was conceived, it immediately became a part of the family and then a part of the black community. Formal adoption was rarely mentioned, except in extreme situations. When necessary, the child was often informally adopted by a member of either the mother's or father's family or by another black family. Historically, adoption meant, "give me the child and I will raise it" with minimal or no legal involvement.

THE BLACK FAMILY'S WILLINGNESS TO SELF-DISCLOSE

Black family loyalty, and support against intrusion by outsiders–especially by non-blacks–is practically a cultural given. Even positive information concerning family members may only be grudgingly shared, if at all. The long history of racism suffered by black

Americans has made it legion to refuse to self-disclose to strangers, no matter how helpful they may present themselves.

Reasons for reticence to self-disclose do not always mean that a family has something to hide. Often it reflects a strong need not to be perceived or judged as inadequate or deviant, as well as a need to formally establish an initial base of mutual respect that will govern interactions so real issues and problems can be discussed. The key element is the need, and almost a demand, for black families to receive genuine respect from outsiders.

These guidelines apply to intervention with any family from any cultural group. However, for the black American family experiencing difficulty, there is probably a keen understanding of what the American "ideal" family is supposed to be like, garnered from personal experiences, television, novels, movies, and even public education. Black family members probably adopt a perspective that these stereotypes form the standard by which they will ultimately be judged. Their consequent experiences are paradoxical: They simultaneously aspire toward and yet reject the artificial standard imposed upon them; they appreciate their own survival skills while feeling helpless to modify their own system; they value persons whom they feel genuinely wish to assist, while rejecting these same persons for daring to judge them; and they openly wish to express their possible current dilemmas while experiencing signal anxiety at the prospect of having self-disclosure utilized as a basis of disrespect and condescension.

Given these paradoxes, the family's initial solutions to developing working relationships include avoidance of the outsider, total or only minimal disclosure, or deceiving the outsider. Black families may self-disclose, while psychologically disenfranchising the outsider in the interest of maintaining self-esteem, thereby negating any meaningful intervention efforts. Or finally, they take a risk with the hope that the practitioner has at least minimal awareness of the cumulative effects of racism. If the latter is true, the worker may be seen as having that rare sensitivity that is so important when building rapport that consists of mutual respect and openness. Hence, each party can acknowledge problem behaviors and attitudes that mitigate against meaningful living and positive family survival.

PATTERNS OF BLACK FAMILY LIFE IN THE 1980s

Changes are occurring swiftly in our society today. An increasing delay in marriage and childbearing is being countered by exponentially rising numbers of adolescent parents. Teen parenting has had a significant impact on marital and family patterns of many Americans. There are an estimated 1.3 million children living with adolescent mothers and an estimated 1.6 million children under the age of five living with mothers who were teenagers when the children were born (Alan Guttmacher Institute, 1981).

Until recently, parenthood in adolescence was considered solely a women's issue, with the adolescent father being viewed as a "shadowy, unknown figure, more a culprit than a potential contributor to either the mother or his offspring" (Joe & Yu, 1984). Traditionally, the father's role–irrespective of his age–has received little attention from social scientists, legal or health care institutions, and policy makers. To a significant extent, services and research in areas of sexual behavior, pregnancy, and parenting have concentrated on teenage females. Despite evidence that successful pregnancy prevention programs for adolescents must include males, a survey showed that a majority of cities in the U.S. have special programs for pregnant teenagers but only one-quarter provide services to male partners (Wallace, Weeks, & Medina, 1982).

In a broader context, adolescent pregnancy and parenting concerns have been one of the primary issues in the black community for the 1980s. In 1978, it was estimated that nearly 12 million teenage men and women were sexually active, and that on the average, teenagers begin sexual activity around age 16 (Alan Guttmacher Institute, 1981). It is the exception to find a young person who has not had premarital intercourse by age 19 (Zelnik & Kantmer, 1980). Teen sexuality and pregnancy have become national concerns in the United States for both the white and black communities.

In the United States, and particularly in poor black communities, the incidence of unintended teenage pregnancy and parenthood has reached epidemic proportions. If current trends continue, four out of ten 14-year-old adolescents will get pregnant at least once by the time they are 20. Nationally, black adolescents account for only

14% of the adolescent population, but 28% of all births to adolescents and 47% of all births to unmarried adolescents are to black teens. In Roxbury and North Dorchester, the adolescent pregnancy rate is two times greater than the city of Boston as a whole.

The consequences of adolescent parenthood are momentous. The drop-out rates from school are significant: 80% of adolescent mothers do not finish high school. Eighty percent of school-age mothers are unmarried and likely to become dependent on an inadequate welfare system. These young women need every service possible to raise their children and still be allowed to be teens and to be prepared for adulthood.

Further, adolescent fathers have been excluded by service providers in the past, and the overall valuing of the father and the male in general are in question. Fathers and potential fathers, who could literally be the adolescent entire population, need much more attention. The notion, of course, is to stress responsibility in these young men, to deal with the issues of frustration, tension, and violence. We also have to bring in role models, and there are individuals who can talk about their profession, share their ideas, and share some of their experiences. For instance, it can be a big deal to have an opportunity to go to someone's office, if that someone happens to be a black male. To hear the term "Mr." or "Doctor" provides an aura of commitment and carries a certain amount of status. We also want to bring in males who are active in the community and carry the title and status of father.

Boston is a microcosm of struggle for many blacks. Most of Roxbury and North Dorchester is characterized by economic deprivation, poor housing, a mixture of over-crowding and loneliness, family breakdown, insufficient educational opportunity, personal disability, and financial instability (Perkins, 1980). Unemployment and underemployment are rampant. A 1975 unemployment survey indicated that Roxbury ranked second highest in unemployment for all of Boston, while North Dorchester ranked seventh, out of a total of 15 communities.

These problems associated with teen sexual activity and pregnancy are felt even more profoundly in the black community since it is essentially a young population. In 1980, the median age for blacks was 25 compared to 31 for whites (Zelnick & Kantmer,

1980). Nationally, 22% of the black population was in the 15-24 age group compared to 18% for whites (National Urban League, 1983).

Further, the percentage of sexually active, never-married black teen women rose from nearly 15% in 1971, to 65% in 1979. The largest increase occurred at one of the most vulnerable ages–15. More than half of every 1,000 black births in 1980 were illegitimate; the overall rate was higher for blacks than in recent earlier periods (U.S. Census, 1983).

Marital stability for adolescents and blacks in general has been influenced by economic and cultural forces. These has been a marked increase in the divorce rate for blacks. For instance, for white women under the age of 30, the chances are nearly two out of four that their marriage will end in divorce, while for black women, the chances are two out of three.

Among the primary variables that influence family life are education, employment, and income. Looking at the 1980 census, we find some progress in certain area for black families yet little change in their status compared with that of white families. The staggering problems of poverty and unemployment remain unchanged for many black families. In education, the proportion of blacks graduating from high school increased slightly, but blacks were still more likely than whites to drop-out. The median number of school years completed by black Americans over 24 years of age was 12.0 in contrast to 12.3 for white Americans (U.S. Census, 1983).

A clearer picture of education for blacks and minorities in general is revealed from Boston data. Forty-seven percent of Boston public school students are black; 28% are white; 17% are Hispanic; and 8% are Asian. Of 57,000 students in the schools, about 75% come from single-parent households or foster homes. Thirty-eight percent of the children come from families on welfare. Nearly 70% of the students come from families whose annual income is less than $20,000 and a third live in homes where the income is under $10,000. Perhaps the most alarming statistic is that, of all students who start high school in Boston, 48% drop out of school before graduation. Of those remaining in high school, one out of every six students is on probation for having committed some type of crime. At some high schools, headmasters estimate that as many as a third of their students have a probation officer (Kenney, 1985).

Employment for blacks provides an important stimulus to the black family. Unemployment has reached critical proportions since 1981, but historically this is nothing new. For young black males, unemployment estimates were as high as 56% in 1980. The unemployment rate for blacks in 1982 was at its highest level since 1945. Overall, 18.9% of blacks were officially unemployed compared to 8.6% for whites. In the years 1972-1982, black unemployment increased from 10.3 to 18.9%. Furthermore, this increase in unemployment during that ten-year period was highest among married black men who were the primary breadwinners.

Just as significant is the unemployment rate of black male teenagers. About 50% of that group was unemployed, compared to 20.4% of white male teenagers. The highest unemployment rates in the country are among black male teenagers in low-income areas of central cities. Their unemployment rate is about 65% and has risen as high as 57% (U.S. Census, 1983).

The rate of teen unemployment is estimated to be more than twice the rate of the general population. Thus a majority of working-age black males fail to achieve the fundamental need of employment. After analyzing economic and census data, Joe and Yu (1984) concluded that 46% of the 8.8 million black men of working age were not in the labor force. Moreover, based on 1982 statistics, the study found that 1.2 million black men were unemployed; 1.8 million had dropped out of the labor force; 186,000 were in prison; and 925,000 were classified as "missing" because the Census Bureau could not locate them (Joe & Yu, 1984).

Jobs for black youth and adults have become scarce through shifts in the labor market, especially in low-wage areas of the country. Many jobs that were once filled by young adolescents are now filled by adults.

Census figures indicate that the 1970s saw little significant change in the socioeconomic status of black families. An increase in educational attainment has produced little in economic benefits for most blacks. Based on the rate of progress in integrating blacks in the labor force in the past decade, it will take 9.3 years to equalize the participation of blacks in low-paying office and clerical jobs, and a period of 90 years before black professionals approximate the proportion of blacks in the population (Staples, 1982).

CONCLUSIONS AND RECOMMENDATIONS

The problem of black teenagers having children out of wedlock has been the focus of researchers and the media over the last 20 years. These reports, no matter how informative, help support and reinforce racist stereotypes.

The government systematically excluded blacks from the mainstream by not giving them the right to vote in the South until the 1960s. Without political, economic, and educational power, blacks could not obtain adequate educational and social opportunities. As a result, 90% of the black population was forced to the bottom of the job market as laborers and domestics prior to World War II. With the support of black institutions, including schools and the church, blacks were able to function. The family served as the foundation for the community, and heads of households could then interact with other parents, religious leaders, and teachers.

In the 1960s successful blacks began to move out of the city, in effect, taking money, influence, role models, and leadership with them. In essence, a part of the black urban foundation was broken. Whites also moved out of the city in much larger numbers. These trends left a void in the tax base of many urban areas. Many blacks and whites were less able to transmit desirable values to their children. A partnership between the city and the suburbs needs to be fostered throughout the country.

The real legacy we have is our children. Consider the following example: A study by the Children's Defense Fund (1989) states that "marriage is now an almost forgotten institution among black teens. The adolescent single mother was the exception in the black community of the 1950s." This trend has become the rule. There are ten states in the Union where out-of-wedlock births to women under age 20 comprise less than 40% of all births; in half the states, this percentage is greater than half. The range goes from 28% in Utah to 71% in New Jersey. In the District of Columbia, the number is 88%. Until recently, adolescent pregnancy has been viewed solely as a black problem. However, the rate of teenage pregnancy among whites is now higher than the rate among blacks. To develop reasonable solutions, we must stop viewing societal problems in racial terms.

The family must serve as the foundation for resolution to the issues affecting blacks today. A partnership must be developed between urban and suburban areas. Many blacks live in the suburbs but work in the city. Urban and suburban churches could work together on projects to enhance community responsiveness to problems blacks face.

Numerous urban areas have teen-parenting programs. Some of these programs stress parenting and responsibility. Thus the retention rate for adolescent mothers is low. Many of these young parents cannot read or write adequately enough to find meaningful employment. If these young parents are going to be successful, they must be able to compete in the marketplace. The focus should be on skill development first and parenting second.

The key to success in this world is education. Increased black community visibility in schools–particularly by its leaders–is needed. The black community must work with children who are talented as well as those not so gifted. We lose many of our young black children simply because no one pays attention to them. Further, it is becoming increasingly difficult to get minority students into undergraduate schools, despite some strides.

Finally, an important part of the black family is the male. Black men are an endangered species. Much more must be done to enhance their self-worth, particularly when they are young (Hendricks, 1982; Battle, 1984).

With troubling changes in governmental policy, diminishing resources, and a shift to the political right in this country, the future of the family and our children is our responsibility. Some students entering college may need programs to teach or enhance their reading skills.

REFERENCES

Battle, S. (1984). *Perceptions and attitudes of Black adolescent fathers: The question of paternity*. Ford Foundation Report.

Billingsley, A. (1968). *Black families in White America*. Englewood Cliffs, NJ: Prentice-Hall.

Blassingame, J. (1972). *The slave community*. New York: Oxford Press.

Children's Defense Fund. (1989). *A Children's Defense Budget*, Washington, DC.

Elkins, S. (1968). Slavery: *A problem in American institutional and intellectual life*. Chicago: University of Chicago.

Franklin, John Hope. (1970). *From slavery to freedom: A history of Negro Americans*. New York: Random House.

Frazier, E. (1939). *The Negro family in tile United States*. Chicago: University of Chicago Press.

Gutman, H. (1976). *The Black family in slavery and freedom, 1750-1925*. New York: Pantheon.

Alan Guttmacher Institute. (1981). *Teenage pregnancy: The problem that hasn't gone away*. New York: Alan Guttmacher Institute.

Hendricks, L. (1982). Unmarried Black adolescent fathers' attitudes toward abortion, contraception and sexuality: A preliminary report. *Journal of Adolescent Health Care*, Vol. 2, 199-203.

Joe, T. & Yu, P. (1984). The "flip side" of Black families headed by women: The economic status of Black men. *The Center for the Study of Social Policy*. Washington, DC.

Kenney, C. (1985). A man with a king-sized job ahead. *Boston Globe*.

The National Urban League. (July, 1983). *Blueprint for action*. Washington, DC.

Perkins, M. (1980). *Population aged 12-19 in Boston neighborhoods, 1980*. Boston: Division of Statistical Data, Boston City Hospital.

Staples, R. (1982). *Black masculinity: The Black male's role in American society*. San Francisco: The Black Scholar Press.

Staples, R. (1981). *The world of Black singles: Changing patterns of male female relations*. Westport, CT: Greenwood Press.

United States Bureau of the Census. (July 1983). *America's Black Population, 1970-1982: A Statistical View*. Washington: U.S. Government Printing Office.

Wallace, H., Weeks, J., & Medina, A. (1982). Services for pregnant teenagers in the large cities of the United States, 1970-1980. *JAMA*, 248:18, 2270-2273.

Zelnik, M. & Kantmer, J. (Sept/Oct 1980). Sexual activity, contraceptive use and pregnancy among metropolitan-area teenagers: 1971-1979. *Family Planning Perspective*, 12:5, 230-237.

COST ISSUES

Medical care resources in the United States are limited–particularly to populations at great risk. It is impossible to respond to all of the perceived needs and demands people may make. Assessments must be made in regard to the amount of resources in the United States that should be devoted to health care. There are two basic approaches in making such determinations: assessment of the marketplace, and thorough planning. Much of our thinking for health care comes out of the culture of poverty advanced in the 1940s, 1950s, and the early 1960s which focused on the purported notion of social deviance to explain social and economic inequality (blaming the victim). The behavioral norms of the poor were viewed as deviant from mainstream American society and as such, formed a social subculture. We still follow this thought process in terms of negative outcomes with the most vulnerable populations. Teen pregnancy, AIDS, and informed mortality are considered conditions that impact the poor, and cost should be controlled to assist them. Effective cost methods for health services will be examined in this section.

Chapter 12

The Context of Health Care Policy:
A Social Exchange Approach
to Cost-Effectiveness

David C. Congdon

SUMMARY. This chapter reviews four cost-effectiveness problems in the United States health care system and seven solutions to them proposed by former Secretary of Health, Education, and Welfare, Joseph A. Califano Jr. (1988). It considers contextual issues of how these problems developed and builds on the proposed recommendations from a social exchange view. Suggested expansions and revisions to Secretary Califano s recommendations are discussed.

In a 1988 discussion of health policy problems, former Secretary of Health, Education, and Welfare, Joseph A. Califano Jr., stated that health care policy is too important to be left to physicians and politicians. He documented a series of cost-effectiveness problems with American health care and proposed several solutions. The purpose of this chapter is to review these problems and recommended solutions in the context of socio-economic forces which have contributed to them. The analysis is based on social exchange theory as developed by George Homans (1950), Peter Michael Blau (1964, 1977), and Richard Emerson (1976). Newly identified issues will be addressed to build on the reviewed proposals and implications, and recommendations will be considered.

Califano (1988) suggests four policy problems with the health

This chapter was originally published in *Journal of Health & Social Policy*, Vol. 1(1) 1989.

care system in the United States: (1) It is less cost-effective than systems in other industrialized countries. U.S. health care achieves similar results for adult patients as systems in Japan, Canada, and Britain, but infant mortality rates are higher in the U.S. Also, this lower overall quality of care costs more than two times the per capita cost in Japan, three times the cost in England, and almost 1 1/2 times the cost in Canada. (2) There is a general discrepancy between diagnosis and corresponding treatment in the medical profession. Califano suggests that it is not likely that these differences are due to a wide variety in training since medical school curricula are largely standardized and there are relatively few (less than 130) schools of medicine in the United States. It is suggested that ill-trained or unethical, purely profit-motivated health care providers may prescribe more expensive than necessary treatment which is often also more intrusive on the patient. An example would be open heart surgery instead of equally effective medication to treat the same problem. (3) Califano documents his experience at Chrysler Corporation where hourly workers take off more time for the same medical problems than do salaried workers. He questions why these circumstances occur. (4) He expresses the need for ongoing advances to address growing problems in health care for such groups as the elderly who have often been neglected. He notes that inadequately researched problems such as incontinence for senior citizens limit their ongoing involvement as productive people who would otherwise require a lower, less costly level of care than if successful treatments were available.

Seven solutions were proposed for these four problems. Regarding overall cost-effectiveness, the Secretary suggested an improvement in quality standards to assure that treatment forms and expenses are both appropriate and not more extensive than they need to be. This would include such measures as treating certain heart conditions with medication, when possible, rather than open heart surgery. It would also include a prescribed length of treatment for particular diagnoses similar to those recommended in diagnostic related group regulations for inpatient care. These could serve as guidelines for a realistic length of time to take off from work for a particular problem. Second, he recommended a cap on awards to the injured party in malpractice decisions, and the elimination of basing attorneys' fees on a percentage of the judgement amount. He argues that these costs are built-in to health care fees. Third, he suggested procedures to screen-out inadequate and unethical providers who may inappropriately diagnose patients; use unnecessary, high cost treatments because of their lack of knowledge or desire to increase profits; and, as a result, raise the number and award amounts of malpractice cases. Fourth, it is acknowledged that some unconventional efforts at treatment should be allowed to continue to promote creativity in developing new, more effective procedures, the strength of American medical practice. Fifth, as a way to save costs in routine health care while allowing for high expenditures when needed, Califano suggested that people need to be better educated about the benefits of preventive care. Sixth, he proposed that answers to continuing large scale problems such as drug abuse and dependency causing illnesses for older citizens require expanded research. Seventh, the Secretary saw these solutions as requiring an increased commitment on the part of health care consumers and the general electorate to demand more cost-effectiveness and a higher quality of services from health care providers. This recommendation argues for placing policy development more in the hands of those who receive and pay for health care than only under the control of physicians and politicians. A social exchange perspective can be helpful in determining the adequacy of these recommendations to address the noted problems.

COMPETITIVE MARKETS IN HEALTH CARE

An introduction to the impact of economic policies on competition in health care is in order before beginning the social exchange analysis. The economics of health care in the United States shares some basic contradictions with other industrial sectors of our neoclassical economic system. Health care purportedly functions in a "free market" system in which, according to Adam Smith (1937), the supply of qualified health care providers will automatically match the demand for health care according to "laws" of the market. Smith's classical economics envisaged a world of consumers who all had the resources to purchase what they required and a world free of monopolies.

He saw monopolies as destructive to the free market system because they would reduce competition among health care providers. Such monopolies would also prohibit some providers from competing at all. As a result, prices would be higher, and the level of care would be less than in a more competitive environment. Many poor people would not be able to afford necessary treatment.

Currently popular neoclassical revisions of Smith's theory allow for monopolistic centralization of power and profit in industry and in the provision of health care. Medical care facilities have often become "big business" and their directors have enjoyed very high salaries. Physicians are considered an elite class in the United States. The importance of their work in saving lives has been transferred to their receiving higher incomes than the average citizen. The average annual net income for practicing physicians in the United States is $78,000 per year compared to a $14,628 gross income average for all workers (Lidz & Perrin, 1987; U.S. Dept. of Commerce, 1987). In a social system which demonstrates its value on occupational functions with financial rewards, that is, perhaps, as it should be. The problem with financial rewards as a valuing mechanism for meritorious service is that they also become their own rewards. Wealthy people accrue power and can monopolistically manipulate markets to accrue more power. For example, the power of physicians could be used to limit enrollment in schools of medicine in the United States so as to reduce the supply of physicians and keep the per capita demand and price for their services high. Also, as Califano suggests, relatively autonomous, and therefore powerful, physicians could prescribe more costly than necessary procedures to assure high profits. While it is important to reward health care providers commensurate with the level at which we value their life-sustaining efforts, it is also important to limit their ability to monopolize health care in a way which imposes unnecessarily expensive treatment on patients or denies treatment to some individuals. These dual goals can be achieved through changing the structure of health care funding and delivery systems so that consumers are: more involved in determining policy and practice, have equal financial status with higher paid health care providers, and will use the opportunity for increased input to take more responsibility for their own health care.

George Homans (1950) has conceptualized activity with others as the basic social exchange process. It is the building block for social involvement, developing a sense of equality and trusting social contact, and the subsequent development of social norms and formal rules for social interaction. Richard Emerson (1976) enhanced the activity construct by conceptualizing it as a single unitized interaction made up of the mutual exchange of resources between two people. From this theoretical foundation, it can be inferred that involving patients and prospective patients in the development of health care policy involves more than their receiving medical care, advice, and education from providers, employers, and other people in positions of power. Involvement also requires that health care providers and other traditionally powerful people, such as employers, also receive advice and education from consumers.

It was Homans' (1950) contention that as people are engaged in social exchange activity, they increasingly perceive each other as equal to themselves. This proposition suggests that problems of alienation in health care, which result from responding only to the concerns of those in positions of power (many providers and employers), could be alleviated by structural changes which require increased attention to the concerns of consumers. As long as money is used to reward the valued work of health care providers, however, increased equality requires that large differences between the high incomes of health care providers and lower incomes of average consumers be reduced. Hawkins (1977) suggests that a truly egalitarian society must have different income or status levels to promote our interest in valuing each other as equal. Rawls (1971) adds that though an equal society will consist of different status levels among which people will move, it must also guarantee that each person has the ability to move from the lowest status level to the highest with reasonable effort. Clearly, many current health care consumers could not realistically achieve the status of providers.

Increased equality of interaction among health care providers and consumers could be approached, economically, through such efforts as limiting top incomes in the health care field and significantly raising the real income of the poorest consumers through increases in the minimum wage and guaranteed opportunities for employment. In order to keep the most talented minds in the health care field, it would be necessary to limit incomes in all fields of endeavor so that there would not be an economic reason to give up medical practice to attain higher incomes elsewhere. In Japan, the ratio of income between the top and bottom 10% of earners is 5 to 1 and per capita health care costs are half as much as in the United States. In the U.S., this ratio is 11 to 1 (Marshall, 1987). Similarly, more cost-effective systems in Canada and England surface in the context of policies which do more to empower the average consumer in relation to providers.

Reduced income and status differences between more economically dominant policy developers and less powerful consumers would result in increased competition among health care providers to meet patient needs. Economically empowered, better informed consumers will more likely move from one health care setting to another to improve the quality of health care they receive. This increased selectivity would encourage providers to improve their quality of care for a competitive price. Theoretically, Blau (1977) has suggested that as people are more equal with others, they will have more opportunity for social contact with them. This social contact would allow consumers to know health care providers better and to know, perhaps, that if they are not receiving what they want from the health care system, they can act to change it or become part of it as physicians or other providers. The opportunities allowed by reduced income differences could promote an environment less dominated by monopolies, allowing competition to function to meet the needs of consumers in the health care field more nearly in the way that Adam Smith projected. These opportunities for increased interaction also allow for increased trust in health promoting relationships.

TRUSTING PROFESSIONAL RELATIONSHIPS

Blau (1964) suggests that trusting social contacts are developed through a process of reiterated social exchanges in which two people learn that their expectations of the other will be fulfilled. As health care consumers are able to move from one provider to another and finally settle on one who meets their expectations, they can begin to trust that provider to meet their needs, not cause them undue trauma, and not prescribe unnecessarily expensive procedures. Similarly, a health care provider, in an egalitarian environment of increased social access and economic opportunities for consumers, should be better able to trust that consumers will follow through with health promoting activities in the prevention and treatment of disease based on the increased awareness and involvement in health care which increased opportunities for involvement have afforded them. Positive consumer steps may include behaviors such as reduced smoking or really resting when treatment calls for it. Beyond the arena of the direct helping relationship, employees who have a trusting relationship with their employers can be increasingly trusted to take off only the time that is needed for an illness without maximizing their use of allowed sick time under an antagonistic labor agreement. In the same way, employers should be able to be trusted to respond to both legitimate health needs of their employees as well as to the goals of the work organization. Although these outcomes may sound idealistic, worker productivity results in environments where trust levels among employees and employers are high have been shown to be much higher than where trust levels are low (Ouchi, 1981; Peters & Waterman, 1982; Marshall, 1987). Less potential for high wage differences among health care providers would promote more effective collegial efforts to solve health care problems and promote prevention. As high profits are limited and the medical profession continues to be valued with higher than average wages, providers will be able to more comfortably focus on delivering high quality services rather than on building empires of financial power. This environment would likely contribute to cultural attitudes that promote health.

COLLECTIVE HEALTH CARE CULTURES

Homans (1950) suggests that as people develop trusting social contacts, social groups begin to behave in accordance with informal norms. These order behavior for the group, allowing the members to coexist. He further postulates that as the group continues to function over time, norms become formalized into a set of rules. These are maintained and change from time to time in order to allow the group to transcend different environmental threats to its existence, and they provide a sense of collective purpose for its members. As health care consumers, providers, and policy setting employers develop increasingly trusting relationships, they have the potential for cooperating in the development of health care cultures which can promote preventive practices and educated decisions about self-care. This education, prevention, and attention to self-care can reduce superfluous complaints and unnecessary use of the health care system; reduce unnecessary insurance expense for employers, consumers, and taxpayers; reduce "down time" on the job for employers; and reduce unnecessarily expensive or physically uncomfortable and stress-producing procedures for consumers. It is important to remember that the drive for excess profits in health care has previously discouraged some providers from promoting preventive health efforts (Katz, 1986). Beyond the cost-effectiveness benefits of lower taxes and insurance payments, increased productivity in the workplace, and less unnecessary medical intrusion in the lives of health care consumers, collective health care cultures have the potential to increase the general social well-being of individuals who participate in them. As people pursue health care as a purpose in their everyday life, they should feel better, be more attentive to work and leisure tasks, and enjoy their activities more fully. These findings imply some basic structural considerations for how to build on Secretary Califano's recommendations.

DISCUSSION

Although the proposals reviewed here all seek to improve cost-effectiveness, when they are examined through the filter of social exchange, the importance of contextual considerations regarding their implementation and final effects is apparent. The need for broadly adopted cost-effective health care standards is basic. Providers and average consumers should both have a voice in determining which standards are appropriate. Health care professionals have a public policy duty to educate community centers about the values of different treatments for their costs until these consumers are satisfied that they are knowledgeable enough to contribute responsibly to decisions about appropriate standards for themselves, their families, and their communities. This duty requires a revolutionary change in the nature of the relationship between providers and consumers so that they see each other as more nearly equal in financial and social terms. This equity can best be approached through increasing minimum wages, limiting top wages through progressive taxation, and guaranteeing employment to all who seek it. Health care standards need to be consistently and continually reviewed, incorporating new information and new consumers in the process similar to the way that many community mental health boards have rotated consumers through participation in making decisions and setting priorities. As many good professors are aware, educating the uninformed clarifies issues for both students and the experts who are teaching them. As consumers become involved in setting treatment standards, they learn from and bring to the process crucial information relevant to life and death issues for themselves or those they care about. The need for increased involvement is nowhere more apparent than in the current dilemma over malpractice awards, insurance rates, and resulting high medical costs.

The American legal system is adversarial. It is anathema to "trust" those against whom one is litigating. Trust, however, is an essential element of improved medical cost-effectiveness in the social exchange view, because it helps patients and providers understand each other's personal and professional dilemmas in the interest of improved health care. It appears that the presently constituted American legal system has little to offer in improving cost-effectiveness outcomes. Perhaps Secretary Califano had this in mind when he recommended limiting malpractice awards and doing away with attorney fees based on their amount, two dominant features of the current system. His recommendations are incomplete, however. If awards are limited, who loses? Wealthy providers don't. They are simply credited with being able to reduce fees because malpractice insurance and judgements are not as high. Also, the negative consequences of malpractice are reduced. Attorneys may lose if their fees are tied to a percentage of the awards. But such contingency plans are discouraged under Califano's proposal. Attorneys would then have to charge enough, on an hourly basis, to pay for the high expenses for talented staffs and conducting time-consuming research. Although the income equity proposals suggested earlier may limit incomes for the highest paid lawyers and increase the ability to pay for the poorest consumers, without high contingency fees, attorneys would probably have to charge much more per hour of service than they presently do. Normal consumers could probably still not afford to pay such high fees, especially if they were not sure if they were going to win their suits. They would be among the losers. Wealthy consumers could afford to risk high attorney fees to win a suit, but they might be discouraged by lowered maximum awards (Califano's proposal may work in their case). Poor and middle-income consumers, the bulk of the citizenry, lose under Califano's malpractice recommendation. It would be more helpful to take medical issues out of the already nontrusting legal system and spend the time and money required to assure a quality system through intensified cost-effectiveness reviews. Compensatory awards could then be adjudicated within the review system. Consumer reviewers would be more likely to give equal consideration to both parties in malpractice concerns if the traditional status inequality between most claimants and providers were reduced and the reviewers saw themselves as more nearly equal with both parties. This equity would tend to remove confounding effects of status bias in making sound review decisions. Also, knowledgeable citizen reviewers would be well prepared to make decisions about the nature of quality in medical care and appropriate consequences for not providing it. This same system could act to screen out inadequate health care providers in malpractice cases and in other regular professional reviews which evaluate provider behavior. An issue underlying intensified community involvement concerns the degree to which the field of medicine could advance if it were restricted by the significant responsibilities for educating consumers and responding to their voice in determining practice.

Free-wheeling, individualized progress has been the driving force behind much of what has built the economy of the United States. An historical perspective suggests that American profitability has been tied to the exploitation of material and human resources ranging from minerals, forests, and productive farm land to immigrant and slave labor (Bowles, Gordon, & Weisskopf, 1983; Katz, 1986; Kuttner, 1984). High profits from these exploits have, in turn, funded high cost research and medical advancement. The

United States faces the depletion of some material resources and the necessary empowerment of its people required to survive in a world where more egalitarian collective policies are showing superiority in generating economic and medical productivity. The involvement of better educated citizens can act to not only raise standards but to relate research advances more directly to broad-based needs. Also, a more equitable distribution of income could redirect the path of medical research away from a narrow focus on maximizing profitability through serving only the very wealthy to more effectively serving a greater number of people. The positive economic impact of broad-based increases in employment levels at higher rates of pay, paid for in part by increased taxes for the very wealthy, has been documented by several authors (Bowles, Gordon, & Weisskopf, 1983; Kuttner, 1984). Economies which support such policies are able to support superior health care to that in the United States (Schorr, 1987). Such a reemphasis would require dramatic changes in United States health care policy. These are possible, however, in an environment influenced more by collegial development models in more collectively oriented cultures. One of the collective concerns we are now facing as a nation is the problem of persistent, dependency producing physical ills which older people are experiencing as they live longer.[1]

A by-product of a health care system driven by the high profits available in complex procedures and research advances is that development is skewed to the areas of practice where money is plentiful. As people with AIDS were found to be wealthy, creative, and valued citizens efforts to fund additional research on this terrible disease were enhanced. The lack of a voice for middle class and poor people in setting health care policy may explain why attention to everyday concerns such as reducing infant mortality lag behind those in smaller, more collectively oriented, industrialized countries.

Secretary Califano talks about the need for increased self care in the United States. At the same time, he does not mention the necessary requirements outlined here to give people a voice in determining their own care. It appears that he is encouraging people to care for themselves better so that they may be better employees and reduce the insurance burden paid largely by employers and tax payers. The rewards of such a limited approach are diffuse, at best. Workers would be more motivated to care for themselves better if they were better educated; if they had higher incomes, were more involved in the goals of their work organization, and felt they would personally lose more by being absent; if they were more involved in health policy decisions for their communities, and if they saw employers and health care providers less as people out to exploit them for maximized profits but more as people who respected them and whom they respected. As the concerns of average citizens are infused to the process of making health care policy, it may become more realistic to identify and treat serious problems early. If workers were better educated to see problems such as a backache as a possible sign of work habits that could eventually detract from the efforts of the valued work group, they may treat it sooner. Appropriately empowered workers may then be able to participate in workplace changes to decrease back problems for themselves. The pain of an older citizen not able to continue traditionally enjoyed shopping trips because of incontinence problems, for which there is no present, adequate treatment, may be reflected and responded to earlier when policy making involves average citizens. These people, who experience such concerns themselves or, on the part of their parents or others they care about, would have a stronger policy voice under the expanded proposals discussed here.

Secretary Califano appropriately cites the importance of letting the people decide about health care policy in the United States. This recommendation is the core of the social exchange approach which I have unfolded here. I have outlined some of the dramatic changes which would be required in order to attain the improved health care cost-effectiveness suggested by these proposals. Mr. Califano's recommendations may yield disappointing results if they are approached without attending to some of the underlying social and economic environmental constraints which have been outlined here. Too often, positive policy recommendations have had limited effect and discredited their authors because they have addressed symptoms of problems without confronting underlying causes. The approach discussed here is designed to shore up the recommendations put forward by the Secretary to provide additional clarity in forming health care policy to enhance cost-effectiveness.

NOTE

1. An extensive discussion of how privileged classes function to dominate and control those in lower classes is offered in Samuel Bowles and Gintis, H. (1986). *Democracy & Capitalism: Property, Community, and the Contradictions of Modern Social Thought.* New York: Basic Books.

REFERENCES

Blau, P. M. (1964). *Exchange and power in social life.* New York: Simon & Schuster.

Blau, P. M. (1977). *Inequality and heterogeneity.* New York: The Free Press.

Bowles, S., Gordon, D. M., & Weisskopf, T. E. (1983). *Beyond the wasteland: The democratic alternative to economic decline.* Garden City, NY: Anchor Press/Doubleday.

Califano, J. A. Jr. (March 20,1988). The health-care chaos. *The New York Times Magazine.*

Emerson, R. M. (1976). Social exchange theory. *Annual Reviews Inc.*, 335-362.

Hawkins, D. (1977). *The science and ethics of equality.* New York: Basic Books.

Homans, G. C. (1950). *The human group.* New York: Harcourt Brace.

Katz, M. (1986). *In the shadow of the poorhouse: A social history of welfare in America.* New York: Basic Books.

Kuttner, R. (1984). *The economic illusion: False choices between prosperity and social justice.* Boston: Houghton Mifflin.

Lidz, R. & Perrin, L. (1987). *Career information center: 7 Health.* (3rd ed.). Mission Hills, CA: Glenco Publishing.

Marshall, R. (1987). *Unheard voices: Labor and economic policy in a competitive world.* New York: Basic Books.

Ouchi, W. B. (1981). *Theory z: How American business can meet the Japanese challenge.* Reading, MA: Addison-Wesley.

Peters, T. J. & Waterman, R. H. (1982). *In search of excellence: Lessons from Americas best-run companies.* New York: Warner Books.

Rawls, J. (1971). *A theory of justice.* Cambridge: The Harvard University Press.

Schorr, A. (1987). *Common decency.* New Haven: Yale University Press.

Smith, A. (1937). *The wealth of nations.* New York: The Modern Library.

United States Department of Commerce, Bureau of the Census. (1987). *Statistical abstract of the United States: 1988.* (108th ed.). Washington: U.S. Government Printing Office.

Chapter 13

A Proposed Cost-Effectiveness Method for Use in Policy Formulation in Human Service Organizations

Michael J. Holosko
John Dobrowolsky
Marvin D. Feit

SUMMARY. This chapter builds on a previous publication and presents additional information on how cost-effectiveness analysis may be used by policy and decision makers in human service organizations (HSOs). It presents a brief history of the use of cost-effectiveness analysis to demonstrate its efficacy in assisting policy makers in a variety of fields. It then comparatively describes two of the best known cost-effective methods–cost-benefit analysis (CBA) and cost-effective analysis (CEA), and argues that the latter is the more appropriate method to be used to effect policy decisions in HSOs. The discussion centers around refining the limitations of the CEA method and proposes a simple model for use in this regard. Recommendations and implications are directed toward managers, administrators, and decision makers of HSOs. Finally, the chapter is attempting to fill a distinct void in the literature in this field and also suggests the use of more meaningful policy formulation and analyses methods in HSOs.

INTRODUCTION

As the human service field evolves from the age of accountability into the age of relevance, never before have human service

---

This chapter was originally published in *Journal of Health & Social Policy*, Vol. 1(3) 1990.

organizations (HSOs) had to respond to their external environments (primarily funding bodies and the public at large) in such precise ways. HSO administrators are continually confronted by the realities of more fiscal accountability, more effectiveness and efficiency and the necessity to develop more prudent ways to develop, implement, and analyze policies. Underlying such demands are two trends which cause additional pressure: (1) there is a steady increase in the demand for social and health services; and, (2) there is a disproportionate dollar increase to meet this demand.

In an earlier article (Holosko, Dobrowolsky, & Feit, 1989), we presented a case for administrators to use a relatively simple cost-effectiveness method (more specifically, cost-effectiveness analysis [CEA]) in order to develop and analyze social or health care policies in HSOs. Indeed, we have argued that one area in which HSO administrators need to evolve is in translating macro-environmental factors into internal (or organizational) quantitative ones for purposes of effecting more informed policy decisions. The purpose of this chapter is to continue in this vein by: (1) demonstrating the importance of using cost-effectiveness methods in policy formulation and analysis; (2) by comparing two of the best known cost outcome analyses methods, cost-benefit analysis (CBA) and CEA; and (3) by proposing a refined CEA method for use by HSO administrators involved in policy decisions. Our main contention is that those who administer HSOs are pivotal to policy and decision making, and require simple methods to assist in rendering such actions in the most cost-effective ways.

I. A HISTORY OF COST-OUTCOME ANALYSIS

An overview of the history of cost-outcome analysis (which includes both CBA and CEA) legitimizes it as a long-standing tried and true method for both developing and analyzing resource, health, social, economic, education, and defense policies. For example, one of the first such evaluations of projects occurred in 1844 with the publication of an essay on *On the Measurement of the Utility of Public Works* by Jules Dupurt. Although the principles stated in this largely theoretical document were used long before, this is generally perceived as being the first known written document addressing CBA (Sassone & Schaffer, 1978). Subsequently, *The River and Harbour Act* (1902) in the U.S., required the Army Corps of Engineers to evaluate federal expenditures for the first time. Later, and with wider application, *The Flood Control Act* mandated such studies and stipulated that benefits must exceed costs (Campen, 1986). This legislation, however, provided no guidelines on the implementation of the criterion for analyses. As a result, many different types of methods and criteria were used.

In 1950, the *Proposed Practices for Economic Analysis of River Basin Projects* known as the "Green Book" was commissioned to establish a generally accepted (and followed) set of criteria aimed at creating methodological uniformity. This document was the first known attempt to ground CBA in economic theory (Campen, 1986). In 1952, the U.S. Bureau of the Budget issued its *Budget Circular A-47* as a guide which lasted into the 1960s. This was replaced by *Senate Document 97* which was primarily used to review plans for use and development of water and related land resources.

Subsequently, theoretical works considered seminal at that time were published in 1958 by Eckstein, Krutilla, and Eckstein, and McKean (Sassone & Schaffer, 1978). As well, throughout the 1950s, analysts at The Rand Corporation, under contract to the U.S. Air Force, further developed CBA and produced a document entitled *The Economics of Defense in the Nuclear Age* by Hitch and Roland in 1960 (Sassone & Schaffer, 1978).

The 1960s marked a rapid growth of research and use of CBA (Ray, 1984). At the same time, CEA was emerging as a relatively new development (Goldman, 1967), although it was generally considered a less thorough method than CBA. (The differences between CBA and CEA will be discussed in more detail later.)

In 1973, a major breakthrough developed with the U.S. Water Resources Council's *Principles and Standards for Planning Water and Related Land Resources*. This document adopted a multiple-objective framework for project evaluation which proved to be an important development in theory and practice of the method.

Although many of these developments centered around water management, CBA made inroads in other areas, particularly in the late 1960s and early 1970s. For example, President Lyndon John-son's planning-programming-budgeting system (PPBS) and the subsequent wave of social regulations facilitated CBA expansion into other areas such as economics, health, education, and income maintenance (Campen, 1986).

CBA gained most of its prominence through Executive Orders by two recent U.S. Presidents. In 1978, Jimmy Carter's *Executive Order 12044* required that significant proposed regulations be sub-jected to regulatory analyses that would identify the economic con-sequences of alternative responses and that the least burdensome of the acceptable alternatives be chosen (Campen, 1986). Similarly, Ronald Reagan signed *Executive Order 12291* in 1981, thereby formally making CBA a control mechanism to his administration's regulatory policy.

Presently, CBA continues to be used in many different sectors of public policy. (For example, see Frost, 1976; Halverson & Ruby, 1981; Gosling & Jackson, 1986.) As well, there appears to be in-creased consideration and use of CBA in the private sector. Evi-dence of this may be seen in applications to employee assistance programs (Myers, 1984; Decker, Starrett, & Redhorse, 1986; Pat-terson, 1987; Holosko & Feit, 1988) and human resource develop-ment programs (Spencer, 1984). It is anticipated that CBA will continue to grow in use in the years to come.

II. COST-BENEFIT ANALYSIS (CBA)

CBA, considered to be applied welfare economics, is generally conducted by using quantitative data only (Levin, 1983). Its pur-pose is to determine if program objectives are economically feasible (Peterson, 1986). To do this, CBA measures benefits which are derived and costs which are incurred in dollar terms, and the method compares the value of benefits to costs (Williams, 1973).

The ability to identify *all* benefits and costs enables CBA to compare alternatives that have different objectives. For example, an HSO faced with several different service problems, but possessing resources to finance a program addressing only one problem, could compare the different alternatives and render a policy decision.

This type of analysis is predominantly conducted by economists due to its inherent complexity, as it involves the identification of direct and indirect social benefits and social costs (Howe, 1971; Mishan, 1973). Moreover, given the difficulty in determining these types of monetary values, tangible and intangible phenomena must be accounted for. As one would expect, these tasks are predominantly theoretically based and often require a great deal of artistic ingenuity (Massey, 1974). As a result, CBA is usually difficult for non-economists to perform.

CBA sets out to answer three basic questions (Peterson, 1986). These are: (1) are benefits greater than costs? (2) among alternative actions, which has the most attractive B/C ratio? and, (3) what is the net benefit of costs produced by this alternative? These questions, and the CBA process are not limited to the initial assessment phase of project selection. Rather, CBA may be used throughout the life of a project because implementation and operationalization often raise new issues which CBA may help address (Ray, 1984).

i. Analytical Processes

The development of CBA has been such that a generally accepted standardized analytical process has emerged. Two variations of this process will be briefly identified.

A simple CBA format is provided by Anderson and Settle (1977). They outline four sequential stages to this method. Stage one is identification, where the task is to identify and list all various effects (e.g., positive and negative) of a proposed project or program. Stage two, the classification stage, entails classifying these effects into economic-efficiency benefits and costs. Stage three is the quantification stage where the economic-efficiency benefits and costs are converted into monetary terms. The final stage is presentation of the findings. This stage is considered to be the weakest link in the CBA process because interpretation of results can be difficult. The primary reason for this is that the analysis is conducted by professionals with economic backgrounds and interpreted by non-economic decision makers.

Finally, Sassone and Schaffer (1978) offer a more comprehensive framework for a CBA process (see Figure 1). These steps include: (1) problem definition; (2) design analysis; (3) data collection; (4) quantitative analysis/social impact analysis; and (5) results. These

FIGURE 1. Cost-Benefit Analysis (CBA) Process

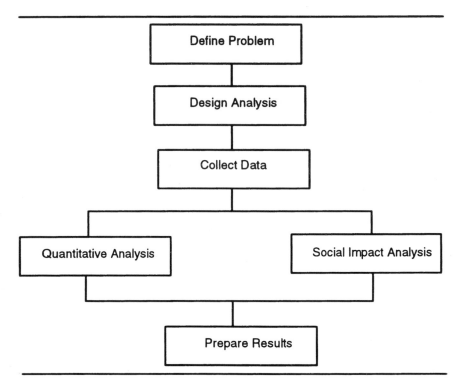

Source: Sassone & Schaffer (1978)

steps involve a planning process which ultimately leads to effecting a decision. By making such information explicit and open for public scrutiny, CBA provides a means of rendering decisions in a more accountable fashion, but the method is not without its criticisms and limitations.

ii. *Limitations*

CBA is limited in that it can only be appropriately used under circumstances where values can be easily placed on benefits, or when values which are difficult to measure are not important (Levin, 1983). It has also been postulated that due to the difficulty experienced with the valuation of intangibles, over-emphasis is placed on readily and easily measurable consequences (Campen, 1986). This has a profound implication for HSOs because many benefits of their programs are extremely difficult to value (Ray, 1984).

Due to the complexity, difficulty, and amount of skill required, CBA can also be very expensive and time consuming to perform (Campen, 1986). Practical analysts, therefore, must perform the minimum necessary to resolve issues satisfactorily rather than to meet idealistic standards for their own sake (Ray, 1984). Consequently, key data may be overlooked. In addition, this suggestion compounds an inherent problem with CBA–poor implementation (Jameson, 1981).

Further, from a political perspective, and due to its inexact nature, CBA may be used to justify predetermined positions (e.g., data may be manipulated to reach predetermined conclusions). Similarly, significant social values such as ethics, rights, entitlements, and due process may be neglected when undertaking CBA (Campen, 1986). It has been suggested that in many instances, for example, CBA does not take into account all benefits and costs.

As a result, equitable distribution of benefits does not happen over the long run. This means that the transfer of benefits from the "haves" to the "have nots" (in an organization or society) occurs at a minimum. To rectify this problem, it has been suggested that weights be assigned to specific groups to ensure they benefit proportionately (Campen, 1986). For example, benefits to a neglected sub-group should be valued lower so that more benefits would be received by them in the long run. In short, these limitations favor options for an easier and more meaningful method for analyzing such data for rendering the most cost-effective decisions.

III. A PROPOSED COST-EFFECTIVENESS METHOD

Clearly, CEA is predominantly the more appropriate method of assessing cost-outcome for human service programs (Anderson & Settle, 1977; Hu, McDonnell, & Swisher, 1981; Levin, 1983; Peterson, 1986; Holosko, Dobrowolsky, & Feit, 1989). Several of the more important reasons are: (1) HSOs usually assess one program at a time and, therefore, use a measurement system that compares alternatives addressing the same objective; (2) CEA is the most effective method known to assess the wide range of intangible benefits found in HSO programs (HSOs deal with human life which is very difficult to value); and (3) CEA is more efficient because it uses data that is already being collected.

Moreover, the process of CEA has been refined to the point where one systematic procedure seems to be the accepted standard (see Peterson, 1986). In this regard, revision of the steps used to perform CEA are not warranted. Nonetheless, its weaknesses need to be addressed.

Specific concerns have been raised in regard to using one criterion in effectiveness assessments (Hitt & Middlemist, 1979; Cameron, 1980; Quinn & Rohrbauch, 1983; Keeley, 1984). Indeed, the possibility exists for programs which offer a greater value for the cost and much more than other program alternatives in total effectiveness to participants (in both primary and secondary benefits) to be excluded because they do not provide the highest C/E ratio (which is currently based on one primary benefit only). The issue thus becomes one of determining how to incorporate a measure that will include primary benefits, as well as secondary benefits, into a standard cost-effectiveness method.

There are, however, a number a constraints which limit the design of this type of method. Foremost, HSO administrators should be able to implement the method with little or no training. As well, the analysis should take a relatively minimal amount of time and resources to complete. Finally, the results of the CEA should be easily understood by decision makers with non-economic backgrounds.

i. Comparison Between CBA and CEA

Measurement attributes are considered to be the most important dimension in both the CBA and CEA processes. Failure to thoroughly and objectively measure all benefits and costs seriously jeopardizes the integrity of any cost-outcome analyses. As such, this has been the area of the greatest debate in regard to cost-outcome analyses, and particular attention has been placed on asses-

TABLE 1. Comparison of Measurement Attributes Between CBA and CEA

Measurement Attribute:	CBA	CEA
1. Uses quantitative data	***	***
2. Uses monetary values for:		
—costs	***	***
—benefits (effects)	***	—
3. Uses unit values for:		
—costs	—	—
—benefits (effects)	—	***
4. Benefits exceed costs	***	—
5. Indicates ways to improve program once in operation	***	***
6. Facilitates accountability	***	*
7. Promotes public interest (in general)	***	*
8. Much of data is easily accessible	—	*
9. Efficient	—	*
10. Measures intangibles easily	—	*
11. Compares different objectives	***	—
12. Values must be easily measured	***	—
13. Expensive and time consuming	***	*
14. Key data may be overlooked	*	***
15. Difficult to implement	***	—
16. Complex to understand	***	*
17. Can be politically manipulated	***	***
18. May not measure all benefits and costs	***	***
19. Data is difficult to determine	***	*
20. Compares one objective	—	***
21. Can account for all effects	***	—

*** = yes
* = somewhat
— = no

sing their measurement attributes. A comparison of the measurement attributes between CBA and CEA is shown in Table 1.

As indicated, CBA uses monetary values to measure benefits and, therefore, can itemize most effects in one way or another. Difficulty is experienced in measuring intangibles because certain values cannot be assigned. As well, the thoroughness of the analyses is time consuming, expensive, and requires specialized expertise.

By comparison, CEA uses unit values to measure effects and, therefore, can only measure one criterion. This criterion, however, is measured thoroughly because its effect, rather than its economic value, is assessed. Moreover, CEA is more efficient and requires less data than CBA.

ii. Alternative Measurement Methods for CEA

The comparison of CBA to CEA suggests that the positive attributes of CBA may be used to offset the weaknesses of CEA. It is difficult to know at this time, however, how an amalgamation between these two methods would precisely fit within the operational constraints of an HSO. Nevertheless, several alternatives emerge from this type of comparison which may contribute to the development of a more useful CEA. Moreover, these alternatives could be easily incorporated in the CEA method previously discussed in the literature (Holosko, Dobrowolsky, & Feit, 1989). The three alternatives involve: (1) multiple criteria assessment; (2) easily measurable benefits with singular criteria assessment; and, (3) multiple criteria with multiple benefits assessment.

1. Multiple Criteria

The use of multiple criteria in CEA stems from the ability of CBA to assess most benefits. Although multiple outcomes are already used to a lesser extent in CEA, they seem to only measure a few positive outcomes. As well, only multiple outcomes of a related nature can be used. What is needed is an effectiveness measure that encompasses as many positive and negative outcomes as possible (an end achieved very well by CBA).

This alternative could be integrated into the CEA process at the step where the common measure of effectiveness is selected (step 4 in Peterson's [1986] method). Thus, rather than choosing one effect, greater attention could be given to analyzing all of the effects caused by the program.

Based on this analysis, the effects with the greatest impact (i.e., on participants, third parties, organizations, communities, societies, etc.) could be listed, priorized and then short-listed for C/E ratio analysis. This would result in C/E ratios for several effects. At this point, weights could be assigned to each effect and, then, the total CEA for each alternative could be calculated.

By way of an example, Table 2 reveals how using the same primary effect to reduce juvenile delinquency, and by using different criteria, actual costs and value to participants shift dramatically. More specifically, by using a program alternative which has four possible outcomes to reduce juvenile delinquency, one primary effectiveness criterion, such as the record of convictions, could be selected. Secondary effects such as the amount of damage to property and the volume of attests could also be measured.

Another program alternative (#2 in Table 2) addressing the same primary effectiveness criterion (i.e., record of convictions) could have different effects than those mentioned above (e.g., the amount of theft and repeat offenses). The issue is, therefore, how to compare these two alternatives, which both possess similar and dissimilar effects. A weighting process, analyzing all listed effects (both positive and negative) could be used to compare the total effect of each alternative.

As shown in Table 2, both alternatives cost the same. The addition of the secondary effects (given the same C/E ratio as the primary effect), and weightings indicating their relative importance, result in different value per participant figures. As a result, the value of Alternative #1 was much higher than that of Alternative #2. The reasons for this are: (1) the secondary effects for Alternative #2 had a lower weight; and (2) one secondary effect for Alternative #2 was worse as a result of the program.

One problem with this method is that it is useful only when the C/E ratios of alternatives are at or near the same cost level. If the C/E ratios have a large variance between them, this method will not provide useful results. With large variances, however, there would be no need to compare alternatives in this way because the lowest cost alternative would clearly be the best choice.

2. Easily Measurable Benefits
with Singular Criterion

Another amalgamation of CBA with CEA is to incorporate easily measurable benefits with one criterion. This alternative involves con-

TABLE 2. Measuring Multiple Criteria in CEA

Effect	C/E	Weight	Total
Alternative #1			
Primary Effect			
1. record of convictions	$2,000	.70	$1,400
ACTUAL COST PER PARTICIPANT			$1,400
Secondary Effects			
2. amount of property damage	$2,000[1]	.5	$1,000
3. volume of arrests	$2,000[1]	.5	$1,000
ACTUAL VALUE PER PARTICIPANT			$3,400
Alternative #2			
Primary Effect			
1. record of convictions	$2,000	.9	$1,800
ACTUAL COST PER PARTICIPANT			$1,800
Secondary Effects			
2. amount of theft	$2,000[1]	−.2[2]	$ −400
3. repeat offenders	$2,000[1]	.3	$ 600
ACTUAL VALUE PER PARTICIPANT			$2,000

[1]All C/E ratios have been common sized to equal the primary effect because the program would be implemented based on the cost for this primary effect.
[2]The amount of theft actually went up rather than down, therefore, this would decrease the total value of the program.

ducting the standard CEA (with the primary effect) and analyzing as many secondary effects as possible associated with that criterion.

This analysis would include the assessment of direct, indirect, tangible, and incommensurable secondary effects analyzed in addition to the CEA of one criterion. Missing from this analysis would be the measurement of intangible benefits for these secondary effects. A conceptual model of this method is shown in Figure 2.

A common characteristic of HSO programs is that much of the

FIGURE 2. A Model for Analyzing Readily Measurable Benefits with One Criterion

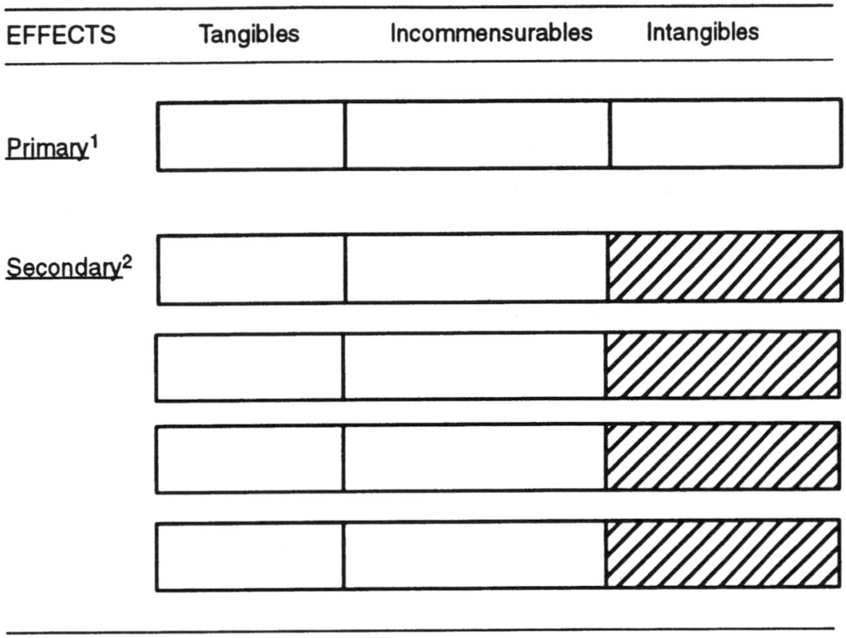

EFFECTS	Tangibles	Incommensurables	Intangibles

Primary[1]

Secondary[2]

[1]Effect measured by standard CEA.
[2]Effects measured by CBA for easily measurable benefits.

☐ = Measured.

 = Not Measured.

effects (or benefits) achieved are intangible. Therefore, even though itemizing and valuing all benefits except for intangibles could be accomplished, lack of measuring intangibles for all secondary effects limit the gains made with this alternative. (The dark shaded areas in Figure 2 cannot be readily measured using this method. As a result, without the data on these intangibles, the compilation of benefits for secondary effects would be limited to a large extent.)

3. Easily Measurable Benefits
with Multiple Criteria

The final amalgamation of CBA with CEA is to incorporate easily measurable benefits with multiple criteria. This alternative is a combination of the first two alternatives. That is, to measure all important effects (primary and secondary) using CEA and all remaining benefits using CBA.

As shown in the second alternative (#2 above), analysis of easily measurable benefits without data on intangibles is not helpful. With this aspect eliminated, what is left is the same method as in the first alternative–measurement of the most important criteria (multiple criteria) in all CEAs. As well, once implemented, it appears as though this alternative would be as time consuming as CBA, if not more so.

In summary, a comparison of the three alternative measurement methods for CEA revealed that each has its own strengths and weaknesses. In regard to weaknesses, it was noted that the analyses of all effects using monetary values associated with CBA was time consuming, costly, complex, and ineffective in measuring the many intangibles found in human service programs.

By contrast, it was shown that measuring multiple outcomes using CEA was an effective method for addressing all effects (an attribute derived from CBA), provided the C/E ratio for each alternative was similar. Based on these findings, it is recommended that the multiple-outcome method be adopted for use in all CEAs.

CONCLUSIONS

The purpose of this article was to develop a manageable cost-effective analysis (CEA) method which could be used to supply policy and decision makers with more useful quantitative information that could contribute to the improved disbursement of resources for optimal cost-effectiveness in human service organizations. It was argued that CEA has been used effectively to render policy decisions in a variety of economic and social programs for a number of years. As well, a review of the strengths and weaknesses of CBA and CEA indicated that the latter is clearly the preferred cost-effective method for a variety of reasons, most notably its simplicity and relevance to decision-making criterion in HSOs.

Attributes from both CBA and CEA were integrated to form three distinct alternative methods for measuring the cost-effectiveness of human service programs. It was found that by using multiple criteria, used in a similar fashion to one criterion in traditional cost-effectiveness analysis, was the best alternative for reaching this end.

Finally, it is our contention that those who affect policy decisions in HSOs can no longer afford to use the FOTSOTP ("Fly Off The Seat Of Their Pants") method. Both funding bodies and the public at large have a need and a right to know that such decisions are being made in relatively rational and informed ways. The sooner such decision-makers adopt such strategies, the more meaningful the results of their decisions will be. Even if they do not change the outcome that much, they will at least be able to be appraised as to how they arrived at such decisions. Clearly, administrators and other decision makers require education and training in the use of such methods.

REFERENCES

Anderson, L. G. & Settle, R. F. (1977). *Benefit-cost analysis: A practical guide.* Lexington: Lexington Books.

Cameron, K. S. (Autumn, 1980). Critical questions in assessing organizational effectiveness. *Organizational Dynamics,* 66-81.

Campen, J. T. (1986). *Benefit cost, and beyond: The political economy of benefit-cost analysis.* Cambridge, MA: Ballinger.

Decker, J. T., Starrett, R., & Redhorse, J. (1986). Evaluating the cost-effectiveness of employee assistance programs. *Social Work, 31*(5), 391-393.

Frost, M. J. (November, 1976). *Cost benefit analysis.* European Conference of Ministers of Transport. Report of the Thirty-Sixth Round Table on Transport Economics. Paris: Economic Research Centre.

Goldman, T. A. (1967). *Cost-effectiveness analysis: New approaches in decision-making.* New York: Frederick A. Praeger.

Gosling, J. J. & Jackson, L. B. (1986). Getting the most out of benefit-cost analysis: Application in the Wisconsin Dept. of Transport. *Government Finance Review, 2*(1), 33-39.

Halverson, R. & Ruby, M. C. (1981). *Benefit-cost analysis of air pollution control.* Lexington, MA: Heath, Lexington Books.

Hitt, M. A. & Middlemist, R. D. (1979). A methodology to develop the criteria and criteria weightings for assessing subunit effectiveness in organizations. *Academy of Management Journal, 22*(2), 356-374.

Holosko, M. J. & Feit, M. D. (1988). *Evaluation of Employee Assistance Programs*. New York: The Haworth Press.

Holosko, M. J., Dobrowolsky, J., & Feit, M. D. (Fall, 1989). Using cost-effectiveness analysis in policy formulation in human service organizations. *Journal of Health & Social Policy, 1*(1).

Howe, C. (1971). *Benefit cost analysis for water system planning*. Washington, DC: American Geophysical Union.

Hu, T., McDonnell, N. S., & Swisher, J. (1981). The application of cost-effectiveness analysis to the evaluation of drug abuse prevention programs: An illustration. *Journal of Drug Issues, 11*(1), 125-138.

Jameson, K. P. (1981). Implementing benefit-cost analysis: Theory meets reality. *Journal of Management Studies, 18*(4), 411-422.

Keeley, M. (1984). Impartiality and participant interest theories of organizational effectiveness. *Administrative Science, 29*, 1-25.

Levin, H. M. (1983). *Cost-effectiveness: A primer*. Beverly Hills: Sage Publications.

Massey, H. G. (March, 1974). *Cost, benefit and risk–keys to valuation of policy alternatives*. Santa Monica, CA: Rand Corporation.

Mishan, E. (1973). *Economics for social decisions: Elements of cost-benefit analysis*. New York: Praeger.

Myers, D. W. (1984). Measuring cost-effectiveness of EAP's. *Risk Management, 31*(11), 56-61.

Patterson, D. (1987). Can a company evaluate the cost/benefits of its wellness efforts? *Compensation and Benefits Review, 19*(3), 63-68.

Peterson, R. D. (1986). The anatomy of cost-effectiveness analysis. *Evaluation Review, 10*(1), 29-44.

Quinn, E. & Rohrbauch, J. (1983). A spatial model of effectiveness criteria: Towards a competing values approach to organizational analysis. *Management Science, 29*, 363-377.

Ray, A. (1984). *Cost-benefit analysis: Issues and methodologies*. Baltimore: The Johns Hopkins University Press.

Sassone, P. G. & Schaffer, W. A. (1978). *Cost-benefit analysis: A Handbook*. New York: Academic Press.

Spencer, L. M. (1984). How to calculate the costs and benefits of an HRD program. *Training, 21*, 40.51.

Williams, A. (1973). Cost-benefit analysis: Bastard science? and/or insidious poison in the body politick? In *Cost benefit and cost-effectiveness*, edited by J.N. Wolfe. London: George Allen & Unwin Ltd.

Chapter 14

Using Cost-Effectiveness Analysis in Policy Formulation in Human Service Organizations

Michael J. Holosko
John Dobrowolsky
Marvin D. Feit

SUMMARY. This chapter describes how decision makers may use a relatively simple cost-effectiveness analysis (CEA) method in policy formulation in human service organizations. The main contention of this chapter is that decision makers need to know how to better effect policy decisions based on quantitative data. CEA is a decision making tool that has been used sparingly in human service organizations, even though it is considered to be extremely useful in developing rational, cost-effective programs for the future. The chapter describes the CEA model in a sequential step-by-step fashion and discusses its analytic processes and how it measures the costs and effects of human service programs. The conclusions and recommendations are targeted at decision makers in human service organizations and stress the importance of obtaining accurate, reliable, and useful cost-effectiveness data.

More than any other type of organization, Human Service Organizations (HSOs), that include health care, educational, and social service institutions, are in dire need of methods to maximize their cost-effectiveness (Halverson & Ruby, 1981; McCrady et al., 1986). One reason for this is that HSOs are under increased pres-

This chapter was originally published in *Journal of Health & Social Policy*, Vol. 1(1) 1989.

sure to reduce costs because they are usually cash users as opposed to cash generators. At the same time, HSOs exist (and are usually mandated) to provide benefits (positive effects) for the people and communities they serve.

A recent article in *The New York Times* that reported on the development of a rating system for measuring the quality of care provided by 300,000 Medicare physicians in the United States, demonstrated this point (Tolchin, 1988). Motivated by concern over the escalation of payments to Medicare physicians, a measurement system is being developed to reduce the costs and increase the effectiveness of physicians.

In Canada, similar studies are taking place. Two of the authors of this article (M.H. & I.D.) were recently involved with a Federal government sub-committee commissioned by the Parliamentary Standing Committee on National Health and Welfare. In their terms of reference, which addressed the development of a model for integrated palliative care for AIDS patients, a major requirement was to perform a cost-effectiveness analysis. The report stated:

> The Standing Committee recommends that a cost-effectiveness analysis be undertaken to examine the model for integrated palliative care as opposed to the present methods of caring for AIDS patients. It is important that the concerns and requirements of AIDS patients and their family and friends be considered in the model. (Expert Working Group on Integrated Palliative Care for Persons with AIDS, 1987)

As demonstrated in these two preceding examples, cost-effectiveness is a central concern to decision makers and funding bodies; and it is anticipated that this trend will continue in many human service systems and their respective organizations.

PURPOSE

In developing and analyzing policy, decision makers are faced with the task of gathering pertinent information that will aid in making the best decision. Generally, this decision making process encompasses the consideration of many different factors from three different perspectives; macro-environmental, internal, and quantitative.

Macro-environmental factors include demographics, lifestyles, social values, economic environment (e.g., competitors), technology, the political milieu, and regulations (Fahey & Narayanan, 1986). Internal factors include management style, personnel factors, and "champions" (e.g., motivated innovators), and quantitative factors consist of short-term plans, research, and cost analyses (Stockslager, 1987).

Clearly, the quantitative component of decision making is one of the primary factors that directly influences decision making (Gordon, 1987). In fact, in regard to HSOs, decision makers are continually urged to consider much more than the "bottom line." Nonetheless, decision makers have developed close working relationships with cost analysts; they consider their input to be of significant value, and use their analyses for a number of important decisions (Sugden & Williams, 1978).

Foremost, and as implied above, cost analysis provides those who formulate and analyze policy with a practical and empirical basis to help make decisions (Massey, Novick, & Peterson, 1972; Sherraden, 1986). Second, the evaluative nature of cost analysis facilitates comparisons among policies, programming strategies, and individual programs (Quade, 1967; Hu, McDonnell, & Swisher 1981). The comparison of alternatives is a critical step in the policy process and, therefore, is enhanced by cost analysis. Further, analysis may be used to control costs (Hoshower & Grum, 1987). Finally, it may be used to justify a policy decision that has been based on many factors (i.e., macro-environmental, internal, and quantitative), one of which is cost analysis (Gosling & Jackson, 1986).

The utility of analyzing costs in relation to outcomes is growing, given the role it plays in the decision making process and the increasing pressure on HSOs to reduce costs. At the same time, however, a deficiency exists within HSOs that generally inhibits the utilization of such tools.

Dobrowolsky (1986) found that most HSO managers lacked the necessary skills in financial and budget management, yet considered such tasks to be important to the successful operation of their organization. As a result, meaningful cost analyses in relation to outcomes are not conducted or used to influence decisions in support of human service programming as frequently as they should be (Hu, McDonnell, & Swisher, 1981; Jameson, 1981).

The purpose of this study is to describe a cost-effectiveness method that may be used to supply those who formulate and analyze social policy with information that will contribute to the utilization of available resources for optimal effectiveness. The intent is to describe a method that can be easily utilized by multi-disciplinary professionals. Our primary assumption is that through the use of a cost-effectiveness method, those who formulate or analyze social policy may be better able to render such decisions in more meaningful ways than they have in the past.

Rationale

By seeking to improve the well-being of individuals, HSOs must utilize existing technologies and methods that have been developed to achieve their ends. To date, most technologies and methods currently in use in HSOs are subjective and qualitative in nature. This means that HSOs usually operate with known processes and unknown outputs.

In the health care sector for instance, the cure of the common cold has not yet been found. Treatment for this illness ranges from mother's chicken soup to complex medication regimens. Conclusive data has not yet been gathered to dispel or promote any one of the methods for providing a positive outcome to cure this illness.

Another example of the subjective and qualitative nature of HSO activities occurs in the social service sector. For instance, methods for improving the plight of the unemployed range from make-work programs to fundamental public policy changes. The absolute outcome of such initiatives, and the benefit they offer individuals and their communities, is not yet known.

In general, all organizations, including HSOs, must relate to their external environments, and overcome uncertainty, so that their missions can be reached. Duncan (1971) explored this further by assessing organizations along two dimensions. One dimension, that involved the number of decision making factors confronting an organization, was called simple (i.e., few factors)/complex (i.e., many factors). The other dimension that involved the degree of change in decision factors in an organization over time was called static (i.e., few changes)/dynamic (i.e., many changes). As might be expected, he found that organizations in complex/dynamic environments face the greatest amount of uncertainty. In contrast, he found that organizations in simple/static environments face the least amount of uncertainty.

Traditionally, most HSOs have operated in environments where there were few major changes. For the past 20 years, however, HSOs as a whole have been moving from operating in a simple/static environment to a complex/dynamic one. There are a number of reasons for this development. First, there is increased pressure on publicly funded organizations, where most HSOs are found, to become more accountable for the use of resources and to use less of them.

Second, with government's decreasing willingness to totally fund HSOs and with increased competition in the for-profit sector (so they seek profit-making ventures in other sectors), profit-making enterprises are developing HSOs of their own to compete against non-profit organizations. Finally, the degree and types of human problems appear to be accelerating at a fast pace. This means that HSOs must monitor the environment and change their missions so that changing client needs can be met.

For these reasons, HSOs have had added pressure placed on them to provide cost-effective service. Failure of HSOs to do so may result in withdrawal of funding, loss of market share, and/or under-served client populations. These results would cause HSOs to close.

By operating in this changing environment, the provision of cost-effective service is not an easy task for HSOs to achieve. As stated above, although their processes for service are generally known, the outputs they generate can be difficult to measure. The dilemma for HSOs, therefore, is to make decisions about outputs that are difficult to measure, so that they are cost-effective for the individuals they serve.

COST-EFFECTIVENESS ANALYSIS (CEA)

CEA is a subset of Cost-Benefit Analysis (CBA) (Anderson & Settle, 1977). A CBA usually becomes a CEA when prices cannot be identified for certain benefits. To aid in this regard, CEA uses unit rather than dollar values to measure end results (see Table 1). Therefore, CEA does not determine if objectives are economically justifiable, but rather, determines if the results of a project are worthwhile (Peterson, 1986).

As with CBA, only quantitative data is used in CEA. The difference lies in the type of quantitative data used. For example, a hospital may use CEA to determine the best way to decrease fatal childbirths (by decreasing the number). By contrast, CBA would monetarily assess whether the benefits of saving children at birth outweigh the costs (Levin, 1983).

The purpose of CEA is to evaluate several different plans (i.e., programs or projects) for achieving a specific objective by weighing costs against effectiveness (Goldman, 1967). CEA cannot be used to compare unrelated objectives. This constraint exists because results of effectiveness are valued in units. For example, alternatives for decreasing fatal childbirths may be compared in units, while decreasing fatal childbirths compared to increasing cancer patients' life span cannot be compared in units.

There are three fundamental approaches to conducting CEA (Peterson, 1986). They are: (1) constant-cost analysis; (2) least-cost analysis; and (3) objective-level analysis. Constant-cost analysis entails identifying and describing the objective, then determining the extent to which the objective might be attained within the limits of the cost involved.

TABLE 1. A Comparison of Techniques Used to Measure Costs in Relation to Outputs

	Technique	Inputs (Costs)	Outputs (Benefits)
1.	Cost-Benefit Analysis	dollars	dollars
2.	Cost-Effectiveness Analysis	dollars	units

Source: Niskanen, 1967

Least-cost analysis involves the identification of the cheapest alternative method to attain the same pre-established level of the objective. Finally, objective-level analysis is used to estimate the costs of achieving varying performance levels under a single alternative.

In the following sub-sections, CEA will be presented in regard to analytical process, measurement of costs and effects, and strengths and weaknesses.

I. The Analytical Process of CEA

Due to the similarity between CBA and CEA, it is not surprising to find that CBA analytical processes have been adopted for CEA. There are, however, several CEA processes that outline more steps than CBA and are more comprehensive in nature. The reason for this appears to be that CEA is most often used by those with less extensive backgrounds than experts in CBA. As a result, CEA processes are outlined in more detail so they can be of practical value.

Also similar to CBA, there is a generally accepted CEA analytical process. Two variations of this process will be discussed.

Levin (1983) outlined nine steps in the CEA process. They are:

1. Identify the problem;
2. List the alternatives;
3. Determine the audience;
4. Decide on the type of analysis to be used
5. Itemize costs;
6. Value costs;
7. Analyze costs;
8. Measure effectiveness; and,
9. Use results.

This process is comprehensive, but leaves the effectiveness measure to the end and is not clear about setting objectives and selecting effectiveness criteria.

Subsequently, Peterson (1986) outlined a ten-step CEA process that addressed the weaknesses found in Levin's model. This process is listed below, and a brief discussion of each of these steps will follow.

1. State the problem situation;
2. Define the objectives;
3. Identify the alternatives;
4. Determine a common measure of effectiveness;
5. Formulate a model for analysis;
6. Estimate and record costs of each alternative;
7. Calculate the effectiveness of each alternative;
8. Perform cost-effectiveness computations;
9. Apply decision criterion; and,
10. Select an acceptable alternative.

1. State the Problem Situation

A clear problem statement should be made to enable the analytical response to be appropriate (Levin, 1983). For example, a school system confronted with declining enrollment might state the problem as "What school should be closed?" To face the real problem, however, the issue is "How to cut the budget in a way that is least damaging to the school system?"

In addition to a clear statement of the problem, its ramifications should also be addressed. For example, by identifying the broad scope affected or potentially affected by the problem, those involved with its resolution may gauge the degree and type of action required. This process also helps in determining the problem by itemizing its symptoms. Usually, the initial problem cited is a symptom of a deeper problem (Mimick & Kantor, 1985). This step is most important in the process because it forms the basis for the remainder of the analysis.

2. Define the Objectives

This step recognizes the difference between identifying the problem and the means that might be pursued to alleviate it (Peterson, 1986). In setting objectives, it is important not to be too limiting (Packer, 1968). Objectives that are too limiting tend to narrow the focus and choice of alternatives. Thus they should be broad enough to encompass a reasonable number of viable alternatives. It is important to note that the objective for a specific problem situation pertains to the CEA endeavour in its entirety and will become the standard by which each alternative solution is ultimately compared (Peterson, 1986).

3. Identify the Alternatives

The purpose of identifying alternatives is to present different means to reach the objectives in response to the problem. This process, therefore, requires a sensitive search for alternatives, one that is usually best achieved by experts and professionals in the field (Levin, 1983).

All relevant alternatives should be identified, then analyzed, regardless of political sensitivity. There are two main reasons for this. First, it is a matter of professional responsibility. Second, political sensitivity may change because it is dependent on many circumstances. Once selected, each alternative must be examined separately in regard to both costs and effects.

4. Determine a Common Measure of Effectiveness

CEA does not use monetary figures exclusively. Instead, effectiveness is measured in both physical and monetary units. In selecting an effectiveness criterion, several criteria should initially be considered and discussed with policy makers and resource providers. Once selected, the criterion should be used as the "common denominator" when the alternatives are compared.

An example of criterion selection is illustrated using alternatives aimed at reducing juvenile delinquency. Possible criteria are: (1) the amount of damage to property; (2) the amount of theft; (3) the volume of arrests; or (4) the record of convictions. Thus, one of these criteria must be selected as the main measure in determining program effectiveness in decreasing juvenile delinquency.

5. Formulate a Model for Analysis

In this step, the objective is to develop a separate budget, or worksheet, for each alternative. An accounting procedure is created so that costs and effects may be recorded systematically. For an example of a CEA worksheet, see Table 2.

Levin (1983) suggests using the "ingredients" method of itemizing costs. In this method, each initiative is described in terms of the resources, or ingredients, used. This results in an account of all resources used.

Three overriding considerations should be recognized in identifying and specifying costs (i.e., ingredients). First, costs should be specified in sufficient detail so their values may be ascertained. Second, the categories in which values are placed should be consistent. Third, the degree or specificity and accuracy in listing costs should depend on the overall contribution to overall costs. For

TABLE 2. Worksheet for CEA (one sheet per alternative)

Costs and Effects	Total Cost	Cost to Sponsor	Cost to Other Government Agencies	Contributed Private Inputs	Imposed Participant and Family Costs
COSTS:					
Personnel					
Facilities					
Materials					
Equipment					
Other					
(specify)					
TOTAL COSTS					
EFFECT:					
Effectiveness Criterion in Units	—	—	—	—	
COST/EFFECTIVENESS (C/E) RADIO					

Source: Holosko and Feit (1981); Levin, 1983; Peterson, 1986.

example, a great deal of attention should be given to personnel costs because they account for approximately three-quarters of total costs in most HSOs (Holosko & Feit, 1981). On the other hand, costs for office supplies should be given less attention.

6. Estimate and Record Costs
for Each Alternative

This step entails the valuation of all costs outlined in the model (above). Here, the costing concepts used in CBA such as opportunity cost and shadow pricing apply to CEA.

As with CBA, this step is of extreme importance because it supplies information to managers, decision makers and policy makers to help account for funds, compare alternatives, and identify the efficiency of current and proposed operations (Hu, McDonnell, & Swisher, 1981). In using cost estimates from various sources, costs should be valued on equal terms. It is important, therefore, to adjust for inflation, location, and the time value of money.

7. Calculate the Effectiveness
of Each Alternative

Not only must costs be estimated, but the results of implementing each alternative must be projected. CEA allows for a direct measure of effectiveness. This is a positive characteristic because it measures an outcome on its own attributes rather than on monetary terms. This is a significant feature for HSOs because most outcomes are difficult to measure and, therefore, lend themselves naturally to traditional evaluation research design. decision makers tend to usually evaluate programs in relation to one specific criterion.

As a result, CEA is less time and resource consuming than CBA. Nonetheless, effectiveness studies still take a significant amount of time and effort. For example, studying the achievement of students in a teaching program may require: (1) substantial testing programs before and after the program; (2) major data-collection analysis; and (3) a significant period of time to plan and conduct the study and evaluate outcomes (Levin, 1983).

8. Perform Cost-Effectiveness Computations

In simple terms, this step entails identifying, classifying, and recording costs, measuring effectiveness, then calculating the cost-effectiveness (C/E) ratios. In HSOs, however, there is a great likelihood that some costs may be inexact due to processes such as estimating and shadow pricing.

To overcome the inexact nature of cost valuation, it is important to consider a range of costs. Stockey and Zeckhauser (1978) recommend the use of sensitivity analysis to enhance the integrity of C/E computations. The purpose of sensitivity analysis is to estimate costs under different assumptions to see how overall C/E figures change. This exercise provides more quality information to decision makers.

Sensitivity analysis involves the manipulation of assumptions underlying cost data. For example, the cost of a health facility center may range from $50,000 to $500,000 depending on the size, location and type of structure. In this case, it would be helpful to produce C/E ratios that are dependent on various costs within this range.

9. Apply Decision Criterion

The effectiveness criterion established at earlier stages in the CEA process is applied to the analysis of the alternatives. Using the criterion as a reference point, a decision is made based on the optimal C/E ratio.

Throughout the analysis, however, more information may be gained about the problem in question that may alter or change the effectiveness criterion used. Managers, decision makers and policy makers, therefore, should be open to the information provided and adjust the criterion as needed.

10. Select an Acceptable Alternative

Finally, based on the above process and previously selected standards such as the objective, criterion, etc., an acceptable alternative must be selected. Peterson (1986) recommends the use of a weighting process that addresses external intervening variables to evaluate each CEA alternative.

There are a number of factors that affect the decision and warrant the use of a weighting process. First, as discussed earlier, the type of approach will affect the decision (i.e., constant-cost, least-cost and objective-level). Second, the amount of funds available during the start-up phase of the program may influence the decision. For example, the alternative with the best C/E ratio may also have the highest start-up costs. If there are not enough funds to meet this requirement, this alternative may not be chosen.

Third, and similar to the second factor, the amount of operating funds may influence the decision. For example, the alternative with the best C/E ratio may also have the highest yearly operating expense. Again, if there are not enough funds to meet this requirement, this alternative may not be chosen. Finally, political issues (mentioned earlier) may be of such great importance that they may negate selection of favorable alternatives.

II. Measuring the Costs and Effects in CEA

The method of measuring the costs in CEA is similar to the method used in CBA because monetary values are the units of input measurement. Concepts such as opportunity cost, shadow pricing, operating cost, private cost, etc., are applicable to CEA.

Measuring effects (or benefits) in HSOs is much more difficult than measuring their costs (Hu, McDonnell, & Swisher, 1981). Due to this difficulty, the use of CBA methods of measuring effects (i.e., in monetary terms) is not completely effective. Rather, the measurement of effects in CEA is performed by assessing units.

As discussed earlier, standard CEA entails the use of one criterion to judge the appropriateness of alternatives. There are, however, several circumstances where this standard method needs to be adjusted. These are in cases of: (1) multiple outcomes; and (2) various secondary outcomes.

Multiple outcomes are instances where a number of objectives may be reached at the same time. For example, a reading program may affect speed, comprehension, and work knowledge. The problem facing decision makers is which alternative is best. Table 3 illustrates this example.

This problem is best faced by using a weighting system (Levin, 1983). In this case, experts and professionals in the field should be approached to identify how much weight each criterion should have. Based on this analysis, the total score for each alternative would be calculated and the one with the highest score would be most appropriate. The difficulty faced by this technique is that all scores must be in the same units of measurement. It does not work well with different units of measurement.

Various secondary outcomes are common to HSO programs (Hu, McDonnell, & Swisher, 1981). For instance, participants receiving drug rehabilitation may reduce drug dependency (i.e., primary outcome) and, also, may develop abilities to gain employment and establish better social support systems (i.e., secondary outcomes). At issue is the identification of all benefits associated with a program, and those associated with other programs. The problem is how to distinguish between them.

In this regard, two research methods can be used to minimize the uncertainty. One is to use multiple measures on a control group (e.g., time series). This method is limited because it is difficult to account for other intervening variables. Another is to use an experimental and control group using a time series. The problem here is that self-selection bias, among other things, may occur (i.e., those who select themselves in the experimental group may put more effort into improving). Although both methods are helpful, they must be used in an operational setting rather than in a hypothetical

TABLE 3. Multiple Outcomes of Alternative Reading Programs

Alternative	Speed	Comprehension	Word Knowledge
A	75	40	55
B	60	65	65
C	85	30	35

Source: Levin, 1983

one. As shown, however, research methods have reliability problems, take a great deal of time and resources, and can only be measured once a pilot project has been operationalized.

III. Strengths and Weaknesses of CEA

The exclusive use of quantitative data makes CEA relatively objective and, hence, generalizable. The dependence on data that is readily available within organizations means that measures of effectiveness should be in line with the ones decision makers normally consider (organizations usually keep track of data requested by decision makers) (Levin, 1983).

By using these standard effectiveness measures, cost data may simply be added (Decker, Starrett, & Redhorse, 1986). Consequently, due to this, less time and other resources are required as compared to CBA. In addition, by using a unit measurement as a criterion, CEA seems a much better means of measuring intangible outcomes.

Although CEA has the capacity to compare projects with the same objective, it cannot be used to compare projects with different objectives. Similarly, a project may be considered to be cost-effective yet may not possess a positive benefit/cost ratio.

Finally, in this regard, the narrow focus taken when measuring the effectiveness of a specific project does not take into account the impact it may have on other projects or the human service system in total. This means that a project may be cost-effective in itself, and yet decrease the cost-effectiveness of related projects. Consequently, there is a distinct possibility that the total cost-effectiveness of all related projects, including the proposed project, may decrease.

CONCLUSIONS AND RECOMMENDATIONS

Clearly, and as this chapter suggests, CEA is predominantly the more appropriate method of measuring cost-outcome for human service programs (Anderson & Settle, 1977; Hu, McDonnell, & Swisher, 1981; Levin, 1983; Pearce, 1983; Peterson, 1986). Several of the more important reasons are: (1) HSOs usually assess one program at a time and, therefore, use a measurement that will compare alternatives addressing the same objective; (2) CEA is the most effective method known to assess the wide range of intangible benefits found in HSO programs (HSOs deal with human life which is very difficult to value); and (3) CEA is more efficient because it uses data which is already being collected. Moreover, the process of CEA has been refined to the point where one systematic procedure seems to be the standard (see Peterson, 1986). In this regard, revisions of the steps used to perform CEA are not warranted.

The CEA method continues the maturation of human service administrators and policy makers in developing appropriate cost-related information from within the field. The uniqueness of this method shifts qualitative data into important and more useful quantitative units for better public accountability.

Some implications affecting the education and/or training of administrators and policy makers are evident. One that stands out is that human service professionals possess the ability and have the capacity for developing cost-related information appropriate for the services they provide. Financial management techniques, that have been an increasingly important component of competent management, will probably be more significant over the next several years. Thus, the CEA and its implementation should pose no unusual burden and be welcomed as a better way of making policy and administrative decisions.

A critical advantage comes with using the CEA. It provides human services administrators with more coherent and rational methods rather than relying more on practice wisdom or intuition. In this way human service managers and policy makers are in a better position to compete effectively with the business approach that relies primarily on cost data. In the long run, human services administrators will demonstrate that they can best manage and make decisions about their field, and the CEA nudges them in that direction.

REFERENCES

Anderson, L. G. & Settle, R. F. (1977). *Benefit-cost analysis: A practical guide.* Lexington: Lexington Books.

Decker, J. T., Starrett, R., & Redhorse, J. (1986). Evaluating the cost-effectiveness of employee assistance programs. *Social Work, 31*(5), 381-393.

Dobrowolsky, J. F. (1986). Administrative skills possessed by upper level managers in human service organizations in southwestern Ontario. Unpublished master's thesis. Windsor, Ontario: University of Windsor.

Duncan, R. B. (1971). Characteristics of organizational environments and perceived environmental uncertainty. In *Organization design: Theory and application*, edited by S. Withane. Littleton, MA: Copley Publishing Group.

Expert Working Group. (1987). *Integrated palliative care for persons with AIDS*. Parliamentary Standing Committee on National Health and Welfare. Ottawa, Canada.

Fahey, L. & Narayanan, V. K. (1986). *Macro-environmental analysis for strategic management*. New York: West.

Goldman, T. A. (1967). *Cost-effectiveness analysis: New approaches in decision making*. New York: Frederick A. Praeger.

Gordon, J. (1987). Romancing the bottom line. *Training, 24*(6), 31-32.

Gosling, J. J. & Jackson, L. B. (1986). Getting the most out of benefit-cost analysis: Application in the Wisconsin Dept. of Transport. *Government Finance Review, 2*(1), 33-39.

Halverson, R. & Ruby, M. C. (1981). *Benefit-cost analysis of air pollution control*. Lexington, MA: Heath, Lexington Books.

Holosko, M. J. & Feit, M. D. (1981). *Workbook for Internal Management*. Knoxville: University of Tennessee–Continuing Education Press.

Hoshower, L. B. & Grum, R. P. (November, 1987). Controlling service center costs. *Management Accounting, 69*(5), 44-48.

Hu, T., McDonnell, N. S., & Swisher, J. (1981). The application of cost-effectiveness analysis to the evaluation of drug abuse prevention programs: An illustration. *Journal of Drug Issues, 11*(1), 125-138.

Jameson, K. P. (1981). Implementing benefit-cost analysis: Theory meets reality. *Journal of Management Studies, 18*(4), 411-422.

Levin, H. M. (1983). *Cost-effectiveness: A primer*. Beverly Hills: Sage Publications.

Massey, H. G., Novick, D., & Peterson, R. E. (February, 1972). *Cost measurement: Tools and methodology for cost-effectiveness analysis*. Santa Monica, CA: Rand Corporation.

McCrady, B., Longabaugh, R., Find, E., Stout, R., Beattie, M., & Ruggieri-Authelet, A. (1986). Cost-effectiveness of alcoholism treatment. *Journal of Consulting and Clinical Psychology, 54*(5), 708-713.

Mimick, R. H. & Kantor, J. (1985). *Managerial accounting and control*. Scarborough, Ontario: Prentice-Hall Canada Inc.

Niskanen, W. A. (1967). Measures of effectiveness. In *Cost-effectiveness analysis*, edited by T. A. Goldman. New York: Frederick A. Praeger.

Packer, A. (Fall, 1968). Applying cost-effectiveness concepts to the community health problem. *Journal of Operating Research Society of America*, 232-237.

Pearce, D. W. (1983). *Cost-benefit analysis*. New York: St. Martin Press.

Peterson, R. D. (1986). The anatomy of cost-effectiveness analysis. *Evaluation Review, 10*(1), 29-44.

Quade, E. S. (1967). Introduction and overview. In *Cost-effectiveness analysis*, edited by T. A. Goldman. New York: Frederick A. Praeger.

Sherraden, M. W. (1986). Benefit-cost analysis as a net present value problem. *Administration in Social Work, 10*(3), 85-97.

Stockey, E. & Zeckhauser, R. (1978). *A primer for policy analysis.* New York: W. W. Norton.

Stockslager, T. (1987). Office automation: Cost justification or management. *ARMA Records Management Quarterly, 21*(4), 15-18.

Sugden, R. & Williams, A. (1978). *Principles of practical cost-benefit analysis.* New York: Oxford.

Tolchin, M. (1988, June 12). U.S. Plans to rate doctors treating medicare patients. *The New York Times*, p. 1.

PREVENTION
AND INTERVENTION ISSUES

In conceptualizing social intervention and characteristics of primary prevention, health providers generally focus on intervention between person and environment in an effort to achieve congruence between the individual's needs and the resources, demands, and opportunities in the environment. Generally, from a broad perspective, there is contact with virtually every human problem. Consequently, there is a need to understand dilemmas that may arise in the intervention process. For instance, providers may have difficulty determining where to intervene in cases such as child abuse, teen pregnancy, and suicide because of the rich detail of individual life patterns. This section will explore primary prevention with the poor, adolescent parents, cancer, and life style characteristics with Hispanics, and AIDS from a policy point of view.

Chapter 15

Primary Prevention with the Poor: Structural Conflicts Between the Health and Welfare Systems

Patricia A. Nolan

SUMMARY. Arizona has developed a Medicaid program under the waiver provisions of Title XIX of the Social Security Act. This chapter examines how well a managed care system for Medicaid recipients works in delivering prevention services. In addition, the conflicts between the welfare system and the delivery of prevention services are explored.

The special nature of prevention services creates significant problems in delivering these services to the poor in American society. These problems arise from the close relationship between poverty and the antecedents of disease: poor nutrition, poor sanitation, crowding, and lack of health care services. The welfare model of delivering services to the poor exacerbates the difficulties of providing prevention services to them. Dependency is rewarded, and a bare minimum of services is provided because of cost and eligibility constraints. Prevention services are intended to be provided to well persons and may not meet the definition of "medically-needed" which is frequently a requirement of health care programs in the welfare mode. In addition, prevention services are low technology services, poorly compensated to the provider.

This chapter was originally published in *Journal of Health & Social Policy*, Vol. 1(1) 1989.

The State of Arizona has made an effort to use a cost-controlled health maintenance model to deliver health services to the very poor. The program, the Arizona Health Care Cost Containment System (AHCCCS), is a modification of the Title XIX program allowed under the Medicaid waiver provisions. The results of this program have not been salutary for many of the people it was planned to serve. Administrative procedures, especially those designed to control costs and determine eligibility, have been so costly themselves that public dollars are diverted from health care services to administration. Some of the most productive prevention strategies have not been supported through the AHCCCS program. Meanwhile, the poor who are ineligible for, or not enrolled in AHCCCS are receiving even fewer health services than before.

Theoretically, enrolling the poor in an HMO-model health care provider should increase the access to preventive medicine services. There are structural barriers in the Arizona version of the Medicaid program that significantly reduce the provision of these services to the poor. These are: (1) the enrollment process, (2) the concept of "medically-required" services, (3) short-term eligibility and mandatory re-enrollment, (4) automatic assignment without regard to the current source of care, (5) significant financial disincentives to providers who actively seek out those in need of prevention services, and (6) the exclusion of family planning services from the program.

The enrollment process of a welfare program in the United States is designed to ensure that only those who meet strict income and asset criteria receive the services of the program. The process starts from the assumption that a person is not entitled to the services. Demonstrating entitlement is time-consuming, demeaning, difficult, and not likely to be undertaken just to get a periodic check-up. Some enrollees in federal welfare programs are automatically entitled to benefits; for example, those receiving Aid to Families with Dependent Children and Supplemental Security Income. These beneficiaries are assigned to provider groups and notified of their enrollment, based upon successful completion of an equally rigorous eligibility process.

Starting with the assumption that a person should not receive the services helps create a second barrier to preventive services. Both the provider and the client operate from a perspective that the client is receiving something for nothing. Since Medicaid is "intended" to provide only "medically-required services," prevention services can be pictured as luxuries by both providers and recipients. The message is clearly communicated that health care is only for the "really sick."

The requirement for frequent reenrollment creates a barrier to continuity of care. The AHCCCS program adds another wrinkle through the provider bidding process: the provider may change because a provider group drops out or fails in the bidding process. This is especially problematic in management of chronic illness, and in the provision of common forms of preventive medicine, such as prenatal care and childhood immunizations. Cultural barriers are more significant when there are no long-term patient-provider relationships. Communication of important prevention and health promotion information is difficult if there is no shared vocabulary. Changing providers can represent so much effort that the client stops seeking care.

The AHCCCS program automatically assigns new enrollees to a plan based upon the bid process, not upon the current source of care. Thus, a pregnant patient receiving prenatal care from a physician when her husband loses his job, may be automatically assigned to a new provider when she becomes AHCCCS enrolled, even though her current physician is an AHCCCS provider. Patients who do not reenroll promptly may be assigned to new providers when they do reenroll.

Preventive medicine is not the practice model followed by every physician. Prevention is not the lifestyle model of many people, including those receiving services through Title XIX. Years of experience in the delivery of prevention services in the public sector and through neighborhood health centers have shown that it is essential to actively seek out clients to promote participation in prevention. Enrolling people in a managed-care program does not assure adoption of prevention behaviors, or even contact with the provider unless severe illness occurs. The financial incentives for active prevention efforts are diluted if the client does not come for services, especially if the client subsequently loses eligibility or is assigned to another group. Among the poor, communication with health care professionals may not seem benign. Going to the doctor may be associated with severe illness or the threat of death, rather than with learning how to live a healthier life. The absence of financial incentives for providing specific outreach and primary prevention services works against the success of the capitation system at the core of the AHCCCS program: the enrollees of this program are not schooled in the practice of seeking prevention services.

The most startling example of these financial disincentives is the decision by the legislature to exclude an important prevention program altogether: family planning services. This decision resulted in fragmentation of care to women, since routine gynecological care and family planning services are combined for most of us. It also results in expensive duplication of such basic health care services as pelvic examinations. In 1988, the legislature remedied this omission, but allowed plans to opt out of providing services for religious reasons. This mixed message on the legitimacy of family planning services may also perpetuate duplication.[1]

Yet, theoretically, "integrating prevention and medical care is less expensive, more convenient, more administratively efficient, and has more community impact than keeping them separated," as Roemer has contended.[2] The model of the Arizona Health Care Cost Containment System fails in preventive care, not because of the capitation model, nor because the prevention and therapeutic services are to be integrated, but because the emphasis remains on the welfare pattern. As long as keeping people off the roles and limiting services to those "medically-needed" is the primary emphasis of publicly-supported health care programs, prevention will not be successfully provided through them.

The AHCCCS program has not lived up to its billing in a number of ways, and some are related to the bidding and administrative concepts built in by the legislature. The delivery of health care through enrollment of recipients with a provider group responsible for primary care and the determination of need for specialty care can effectively deliver both preventive and therapeutic health services. AHCCCS is saddled with unwieldy eligibility and enrollment procedures and with disincentives for outreach and specific prevention services built in by the legislature to control costs. As long as our intention is to restrict health care services to the poor, we will be unable to achieve the benefits of current knowledge about the prevention of disease and the promotion of health.

REFERENCE NOTES

1. ARS 36-2901 et seq., as amended, 1988, and rules adopted subsequent to statute.

2. Roemer, M. *An Introduction to the U.S. Health Care System*, Springer Publishing, (NY) 1986.

Chapter 16

Fostering Primary and Secondary Prevention in Public Policy for Pregnant Adolescents

Peggy B. Smith
Susan K. Kutzner

SUMMARY. The diverse factors associated with sexuality among adolescents and the specific issues related to contraception in this developmentally diverse group result in complexity in policy formation. The future of an adolescent may be determined solely on the basis of access to supportive physical and emotional services funded by public and private sector monies. The purpose of this chapter is to briefly present contemporary and social policies regarding pregnant adolescent health care. Suggestions as to how these policies can be translated into public adolescent health models are provided. The strategies will be related to primary and secondary public policy interventions.

INTRODUCTION

While the absolute birth rate among adolescents aged 15-19 years has declined in the United States during the last ten years, other industrialized nations still report lower birth rates for this age group. The perinatal health and social consequences for pregnant

---

This chapter was originally published in *Journal of Health & Social Policy*, Vol. 1(1) 1989.

adolescents limit and/or deplete their financial power, and ultimately, limit their access to private sector health care services.
Subsequently, these adolescents require health services from publicly subsidized programs. The delivery of such programs is heavily
influenced by a variety of public policy decisions that attempt to
address short- and long-term problems of this age group in a cost-
effective manner. Under optimal circumstances, such strategies not
only assist the adolescent at risk, but are coordinated with indigent
health care legislation. These social and health interventions can
benefit society if policies are data driven and have a strategic plan.
Short-term policies address crises and ultimately result in frag-
mented and limited services.

The purpose of this chapter is to briefly present contemporary
and social policies regarding pregnant adolescent health care.
Suggestions as to how these policies can be translated into public
adolescent health models are provided. The strategies will be related to primary and secondary public policy interventions.

PRIMARY PREVENTION MODELS

Contemporary primary prevention programs focused on children
and adolescents were established as broad-based programs, especially those programs that targeted child abuse and neglect (Howze
& Kotch, 1984). Public policy can be developed vis-à-vis primary
prevention models that, in turn, promotes reinvestment of public
resources in programs that contribute to a decreased prevalence of
adolescent pregnancies. These benefits of public policy initiatives
also encompass an increase in health promotion activities such as
regular health check-ups, and cervical and breast cancer prevention
screening.

Prevention models can generate freestanding family planning or
school-based health clinics. Politically, the actual implementation
of these programs with public dollars frequently faces opposition.
Public criticism of these policies includes an erroneous interpretation that reproductive health policies for adolescents implies tacit
encouragement of premarital sex among minors. School-based
health clinics that attempt to operate under the aegis of a school
district or educational system are "at risk" for public notoriety and

confrontation (Cassell, 1985). On the other hand, clinical services that are aligned with public health and/or academically affiliated health services (e.g., medical or nursing schools) seem to emerge relatively unscathed by community controversy. These programs usually have the support from the professional and lay communities that facilitate the adolescents' access to services.

In spite of the politics and controversies associated with pregnancy prevention programs within the public school system, some creative strategies can facilitate policies to promote primary prevention of adolescent pregnancy and initiate positive self-care health practices. One such strategy is to inculcate policy development within large public institutions such as state health departments and legislatures rather than to place politically vulnerable individuals or groups such as school board members, superintendents, or school administrators in the policy development dilemma. The most flexible vehicle to accomplish this type of policy development is through interagency agreements. These agreements are developed by negotiating and consensus building among anonymous groups of professional and private individuals. The process is a collective and collaborative one that works within a strategic plan to formulate proactive adolescent policies. An example would be the development of an interagency agreement between a health provider(s) and a regional or state educational agency. The agreement might recommend or perhaps mandate health services housed within educational settings and standardized reproductive health curricular modules to be provided in public school settings with linkages to health care settings for a variety of services (e.g., family planning, sexually transmitted disease (STD) treatment and screening, and prenatal care). Within an interagency agreement, professional educators and health care providers can actually deliver critical services to an at-risk group without controversy or harassment.

These primary health prevention policies can also maximize adolescent utilization of reproductive health services. An emphasis on client enhancement strategies such as those historically used in developing countries (e.g., India, South America) is appropriate for at-risk sexually active adolescents. The strategies can include incentives such as health care packets or gifts, or specialized services such as child care, transportation, and recreational activities. The strategies emphasize an adolescent's desired activity or item that was usually unattainable but may, in fact, encourage utilization of reproductive health services.

Incentive strategies can be expanded to encourage self-care health behaviors such as an increased number of clinic visits and recruitment of the adolescent's sexual partner for education and counseling. The policies should be supportive of the adolescent population's needs and evaluated carefully to rule out any perceptions of racial or ethnic coercion. Interpretations of these policies must be supported by key community groups who should also participate in negotiating and consensus-building strategies.

The most controversy related to adolescent pregnancy prevention is the offering of cash incentives for continued family planning participation. An example of this strategy might be a yearly review of quantifiable objectives such as adolescents' self-care activities, number of family planning and/or education visits, and maintenance of nonfertile status. An annual or accrued cash benefit might be offered to the adolescent who met delineated criteria associated with these objectives. These incentives should be offered without perceived or actual negative ramifications such as a decrease in quality of health services or interruption in benefits from public sector agencies. Because adolescents are severely limited financially in regard to the purchase of health services, the policies should never be dependent on eligibility guidelines to access public sector services and on maintenance of associated health care subsidies. Positive examples of this strategy are used in scholarship programs in New York City and support positive outcomes such as good health and educational goals. The program should promote positive self-care health behaviors and not be perceived as a bribe or coercion.

PROVISION OF STERILIZATION FOR MATURE MINORS

Sterilization of mature minors, while controversial, is another prevention strategy. Federal statute and funding guidelines prohibit federal reimbursement for tubal ligation procedures for women under 21 years of age (Johnson, 1985). However, there are mature young women who have several children and have reached a decision regarding sterilization as a permanent family planning measure. Also, this group may include women who must limit the number of children secondary to pathological medical health histories. The provision of state funds as a possible local or regional policy alternative to lack of federal funding for minors requesting voluntary sterilization procedures may be a viable option for this special group of young women. If tubal ligation procedures were available to this age group, perhaps these women would utilize the option to limit family size.

INCENTIVES TO PROVIDERS FOR PRIMARY PREVENTION OF ADOLESCENT PREGNANCY

Policies that enhance self-care health practices in adolescents may be maximized if similar incentives are offered to the health care professionals and/or agencies. Policy initiatives may be realized especially if the incentive relates to financial/economic concerns. Title XX in several states currently places a funding ceiling on family planning for service contracts. Therefore, an increase in monies allocated for reproductive health services to adolescents would be viewed as an incentive to health care professionals to service this group. An increase in reimbursement rates to providers may also increase accessibility of services to limited income adolescents. The increase in reimbursement rates would impact routine services, especially those services that currently exceed the reimbursement rate. This is especially significant with adolescent clients who are generally not treated consistently in the medical community and may subsequently require acute health services and lengthy medical and other visits.

The increase in reimbursement rates would be especially appropriate for specific procedures such as insertion of an intrauterine device (IUD). Current reproductive technology includes two IUDs (e.g., Progestasert and Copper T-380A) that are available to providers. However, the costs of these devices are not covered under most state reimbursement rates. (Note: In 1989 the cost of both devices was $84 plus an insertion fee.) By increasing reimbursement rates, the technology is available to clients and more choices are available for adolescent decision making.

PREGNANCY PREVENTION MARKETING AMONG AT-RISK GROUPS

Primary pregnancy prevention policy can be positively implemented by creative marketing of adolescent self-care health services. Self-care health programs should be appealing to adolescents and have attractive and informative advertising. The program content could include facts about sexuality and birth control, benefits of abstinence or postponement of sexual activity. Currently, most programs are understaffed and delete the educational/counseling components in lieu of direct clinical services. Monies to support education and counseling of adolescent clients are imperative. Increasing and broadening reimbursement rates in adolescent health services will also indirectly support a positive marketing strategy.

Primary pregnancy prevention advertising can target Aid to Families with Dependent Children (AFDC) households with adolescents. Information regarding pregnancy prevention programs could be included in routine mailings to these identified groups such as in utility bills, subsidy checks, etc. The information could inform the clients of the location of health services, the benefits of family planning, and access/transportation to services. This strategy should be based on appropriate timing and frequency of advertising campaigns. Periodic mailings are more effective than one-time efforts because adolescents may or may not remember specific details or lose the materials. If the information is associated with a periodic mailing such as a regular billing or reimbursement schedule, the adolescent may become accustomed to looking for information. If the adolescent is suddenly panicked and in need of services, the materials may be readily available.

IMPROVING ACCESS TO ADOLESCENT PREVENTIVE SERVICES

Policy strategies must have a multi-dimensional approach in order to enhance client utilization at minimal or no cost to the provider. Combining maternity and well-baby services with preventive family planning facilitates the effect of policies on at-risk clients. Complementary services at a single clinical site are ideal for both the client and the provider. An example of a logical incorporation is the combination of EPSDT (Early Periodic Screening Development and Testing) medical screens and family planning examinations into one service contract. Family planning visits could be included with the periodic EPSDT screening services.

Long-term financial paybacks to agencies are significant with multi-service contracts. Family planning services have a larger federal share than EPSDT screening services. The incorporation of these programs into multi-service contracts would shift a significant number of adolescent cases over to family planning funding. The resulting EPSDT savings could be used to screen younger clients and could also be directed to male and female adolescents who are not ordinarily included in reproductive health programs. With a preventive health emphasis on education and counseling, duplicate visits would be eliminated and time and resources would be maximized.

SECONDARY PREGNANCY PREVENTION POLICIES

Primary prevention of adolescent pregnancy is the most cost-effective policy approach. Secondary pregnancy prevention policies must also be developed to serve a smaller group of adolescents. These policies need to be innovative and creative in order to deliver social, medical, and financial services to pregnant adolescents. While it is obvious that a secondary approach cannot prevent a first pregnancy, secondary prevention policies can be effective in preventing subsequent pregnancies, empower adolescents to access educational programs to avoid school drop-out, and build self-esteem and self-sufficiency as adults. The secondary pregnancy prevention policies need to be directed at special school-based prenatal care clinics and on-site child care facilities.

ADOLESCENT AFDC RECIPIENT OUTREACH

Once pregnant, an adolescent has a 60% chance of becoming pregnant again during her adolescent years (United States Commission on Population Growth, 1972). Policies that are responsive to adolescent development and associated behaviors can provide a supportive safety net for documented at-risk adolescent mothers. One policy approach includes the recruitment of private sector participation. The purpose of this collaboration would be to expand the current direct health care staff care to AFDC and food stamp applicants as well as adolescent family planning clients. For example, the utilization of professional nurses educated at the master's level with nurse practitioner skills could extend and enhance the clinical agencies' effectiveness. The ultimate benefit of outreach services on unintended pregnancies may be significant. Educational and counseling groups, as well as individual sessions, may constitute a thoughtful and powerful intervention for AFDC adolescents. Critical information provided in the groups and individual sessions includes reproductive health self-care, emotional and physical sexual development, birth control methods including abstinence, and prevention of sexually transmitted diseases. These outreach efforts should be combined with client transportation to other agencies, aggressive appointment reminders, and follow-up for health encounters. The more aggressive the follow-up, the greater the benefit to the client and provider through decreased unintended pregnancy rates and positive adolescent health outcomes.

Volunteer staff who participate in a thorough orientation program by health professionals may facilitate an aggressive outreach approach. Health care professionals may be able to extend the effects of their services through volunteer staffing of strong outreach, education, and referral. This would also increase the number of clients referred to family planning clinics, increase the number of adolescents who utilize effective birth control techniques and hopefully, decrease their subsequent unintended pregnancies.

SUMMARY AND COMMENTS

The overall objective in averting subsequent unintended pregnancies among adolescents and the ultimate reduction in personal, social, and economic suffering is congruent with a primary prevention of pregnancy policy approach to a serious social problem. The diverse factors associated with sexuality among adolescents and the specific issues related to contraception in this developmentally diverse age group result in complexity in policy formation. And, because of the complexity of the issues related to adolescent health care and pregnancy prevention, policies must be carefully developed within a strategic planning focus. The worst case scenario for adolescent policy formulation is an unintended consequence of curtailed services and limited outreach.

However, serious problems are present among adolescents currently seeking care in family planning and pregnancy programs. Sexual activity among adolescents is a reality and appropriate methods of birth control to avoid unintended adolescent pregnancies are imperative. However, the choice of a birth control method cannot be mandated and must be specific to the individual's physical and emotional needs. For instance, the IUD may offer an effective method of birth control. However, the IUD is recommended for monogamous women. Observations of contemporary adolescent behavior suggest that a large percentage of adolescents have more than one sexual partner. Moreover, an individual with more than one sexual partner is at higher risk for contracting a sexually transmitted disease. Therefore, the IUD may be contraindicated. Reports from adolescent family planning programs (Smith et al., 1988) indicate a STD prevalence among clients of 14-27 percent. The highest incidence of STDs occurs among young people aged 15-24. Therefore, the effectiveness of this birth control method may be decreased secondary to the developmental behaviors of the adolescent group.

The policies formulated for self-care health activities of adolescents need to be flexible, diverse, and creative. The future of an adolescent may be determined solely on the basis of access to supportive physical and emotional services funded by public and private sector monies. Enhancement of reimbursements to providers, development of aggressive outreach services, and creative educational marketing to the adolescent population, supplemented by volunteer labor, may begin to impact adolescent pregnancy rates and health status. While the reimbursement rates may be increased significantly or clients targeted as at risk, entitlement programs such as Title XIX and Medicaid are not current with client needs nor do they aggressively process and reimburse claims from agencies and providers. Policies for this at-risk group of adolescent clients must do more than promote programming. Information systems and development of efficient cost-reimbursement strategies must be developed concurrently with policy groups to measure and evaluate baseline levels of client outcomes and effectiveness of services.

REFERENCES

Cassell, C. (1985). The politics of sex education: Campaigns and crusades. In *Adolescent reproductive health: Handbook for the health professional*, edited by P.B. Smith and D.M. Mumford. New York: Gordon Press.

Howze, D.C. and Kotch, J.B. (1984). Disentangling life events, stress and social support: Implications for the primary prevention of child abuse and neglect. *Child Abuse & Neglect, 8*, 401-409.

Johnson, S.B. (1985). Law and reproductive health. In *Adolescent reproductive health: Handbook for the health professional*, edited by P.B. Smith and D.M. Mumford. New York: Gordon Press.

Smith, P., Phillips, L.E., Faro, S., McGill, L., and Wait, R.B. (1988). Predominant sexually transmitted disease among different age and ethnic groups of indigent sexually active adolescents attending a family planning clinic. *Journal of Adolescent Health Care*, 291-295.

United States Commission on Population Growth (1972). *Report by the United States Commission on Population Growth*. Washington, DC: Government Printing Office, 355-374.

Chapter 17

Hispanics and Cancer-Preventive Behavior: The Development of a Behavioral Model and Its Policy Implications

Judith T. Gonzalez
Jan Atwood
John A. Garcia
Frank L. Meyskens

SUMMARY. This chapter presents the theoretical development of a model that predicts the conditions under which Hispanics seek preventive health care. Research trends show that Hispanics tend to delay preventive care, resulting in higher morbidity and mortality rates for serious diseases such as cancer. Since many serious diseases, such as heart disease, diabetes, and cancer can be prevented or treated more effectively if detected early, it is crucial to understand the motivating forces behind Hispanics' preventive health behavior. The Hispanic model, which is an extension of the Health Behavior in Cancer Prevention Model developed by Atwood (1986), includes as core variables environmental barriers to access and English language proficiency, as well as social support, health beliefs, self-efficacy, or perceived skill, health locus of control, and health values. The practical health policy applications of the model are also discussed.

INTRODUCTION

Many serious diseases, such as heart disease, cancer, and diabetes can be prevented or treated successfully if detected early. Yet current research shows that Hispanics[1] are not receiving early pre-

This chapter was originally published in *Journal of Health & Social Policy*, Vol. 1(2) 1989.

ventive care (Daly, Clark, and McGuire, 1985). Crucial to changing this trend is the understanding of how preventive health behavior is affected among Hispanics, which requires the development and testing of theory that takes into account unique environmental and cultural factors that affect Hispanics' health behavior.

This paper presents the development of such a theoretical model and its policy implications. This model, the Hispanic Health Behavior in Cancer Prevention Model is based on the Health Behavior in Cancer Prevention Model (HBCP) (Atwood, 1986). Preventive health behavior refers to any behavior directed to the prevention or detection of disease at the asymptomatic stage (Kasl and Cobb, 1986). It consists of three components: compliance; adherence to a provider-initiated therapy; and self-care. Compliance results when the patient implements the provider's course of treatment (Basch et al., 1983; Hershey et al., 1980; Watts, 1982). Adherence is a negotiated agreement between the client and the provider initiated by the latter (Hindi-Alexander and Throm, 1987). Self-care refers to client-initiated behavioral change designed to promote health without the provider's direct involvement. Self-care requires considerable independence and decision making congruent with the patient's culture (Pender, 1987). This model applies to self-care and adherence, in contrast to compliance.

This chapter discusses delayed health care among Hispanics and then proceeds to describe the model, to support it with extant literature, and to present policy implications.

IMPORTANCE OF PREVENTIVE CARE

In a cross-sectional study of San Antonio Mexican American and Anglo females, Daly et al. (1985) found important differences between the two groups at first diagnosis for breast cancer. Significantly more Mexican American women over 50 years of age, compared to Anglo women had larger tumors, axillary mode involvement, and showed an estrogen negative receptor status at time of breast cancer diagnosis. Samet et al. (1987) examined cancer survival rates by ethnic group for 31,465 incident cases diagnosed from 1969 to 1982 in New Mexico and Arizona. Hispanic cancer patients were significantly more likely to have more advanced cancers at first diagnosis than were whites. One- and five-year survival rates were computed for each type of cancer. Overall, one- and five-year survival rates for Hispanics were significantly lower than for Anglos. Hispanics were also significantly less likely to have received treatment for the cancer after initial diagnosis when compared with Anglos.

The data clearly indicate that Mexican Americans are less likely to engage in preventive care, are diagnosed later for cancer, delay treatment once cancer is diagnosed, and show poorer survival rates. Data on Hispanic colon cancer rates from 105 Angeles County Cancer Surveillance Program and nationwide (Mack et al., 1985; Proceedings of the Hispanic Cancer Control Program Workshop, National Cancer Institute, 1986) show that rates for Hispanics are climbing. Savitz (1986) presents data showing a 150-percent increase in Hispanic colon cancer incidence from 1971 to 1981. Additionally, colon cancer risk rates (Savitz, 1986) were 0.4 for immigrant Mexican Americans compared to 0.9 for native-born Mexican Americans. Savitz' data suggest that acculturation as measured by years in the United States relates to a higher incidence and increasing risk for colon cancer among Mexican Americans.

Research Inconsistencies

The Health Belief Model (HBM) is often applied to explain preventive behavior. This model (Janz and Becker, 1984; Rosenstock, 1974) postulates that health behavior is a function of three factors: (1) perceived severity of the disease in question, (2) perceived susceptibility, and (3) a balance between barriers and benefits of a given therapeutic or preventive strategy. However, research testing of this model has been plagued with inconsistencies. Kegeles (1963) found that perceived severity of dental disease bore no association with maintained prophylaxis. An earlier study by Hochbaum (1958) showed a positive relationship between perceived susceptibility and benefits and rate of voluntary tuberculosis X-ray screening, lending support to the HBM. Other studies (Pender, 1987; Becker et al., 1977a) also support the HBM. Calnan and Moss (1984) found that perceived vulnerability to breast cancer failed to discriminate between women who performed breast self examination satisfactorily at a six-month follow-up and those who were not proficient, but did predict first attendance at a training class. Apparently, maintenance and proficiency of behavior require other factors not accounted for in the HBM.

Other aspects of health behavior, such as background demographic variables (Sackett and Haynes, 1976; Cummings, Becker, and Maile, 1980; Rosenstock, 1974) health status (Belloc and Breslow, 1972), social support (Gottlieb, 1981; Cummings, Becker, and Maile, 1980), self-efficacy, (Chambliss and Murray, 1979; O'Leary, 1985) and accessibility to health care (Cummings, Becker, and Maile, 1980; Estrada, 1987) have been shown to relate to preventive behavior.

In order to organize the myriad variables previously substantiated as predictors of compliance, Cummings, Becker, and Maile (1980) gathered the related variables from McKinlay's (1972) taxonomy and submitted them to a content validity analysis using an expert panel of judges. Smallest space analysis revealed six unique groupings: (1) accessibility of health services, i.e., physical availability of services and ease of communication with the provider; (2) attitudes toward health care, e.g., health value orientation; (3) threat of illness (HBM), e.g., perceived severity and susceptibility; (4) knowledge about disease; (5) social interactions, social norms, and social structure, e.g., the social network structure and functions; (6) demographic characteristics (Cummings, Becker, and Maile, 1980, p. 137). Each of these are included in the adapted HBCP model.

Hence, the Hispanic Health Behavior in Cancer Prevention Model includes background demographic factors, health knowledge, the HBM, health status, health values, self- and treatment efficacy, and social support. The Hispanic Model also includes English language proficiency, and barriers to health care utilization as core components. English language proficiency and barriers to utilization are not included in the original HBCP (Atwood, 1986). These last two factors specific to the Hispanic HBCP model and their posited effects on preventive health behavior are outlined in this chapter. Figure 1 shows the proposed model.

Model Structure

This five-stage behavioral model is based on a careful review of the compliance and adherence literature and the HBCP (Atwood, 1986).

FIGURE 1. Diagram of Health Behavior in Cancer Prevention (HBCP) Model: Adapted for Hispanic Populations (Atwood, 1986)

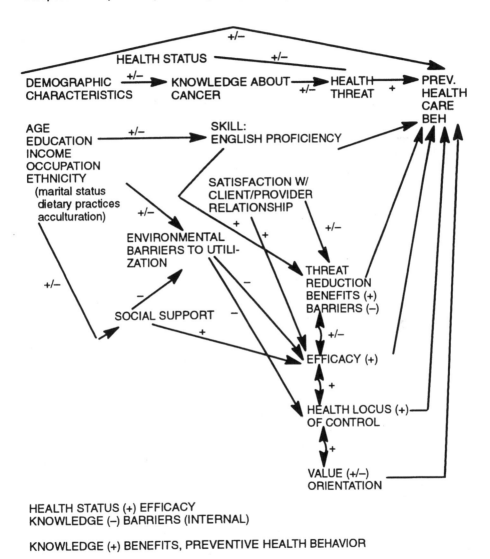

HEALTH STATUS (+) EFFICACY
KNOWLEDGE (–) BARRIERS (INTERNAL)

KNOWLEDGE (+) BENEFITS, PREVENTIVE HEALTH BEHAVIOR

RELATIONSHIPS: +=positive –=negative +/–=unpredicted (mixed findings in the literature)

STAGE 1   STAGE 2   STAGE 3   STAGE 4   STAGE 5

The HBCP applied to Hispanics consists of five stages as illustrated in Figure 1. Its theoretical underpinnings are substantiated in the literature review. The linkages are as follows:

1. Stage I are background demographic variables that relate directly to barriers to utilization, social support, preventive health care, and English proficiency.
2. Stage II model variables are social support (Tilden and Gaylan, 1987), health status (Belloc and Breslow, 1972), and barriers to utilization (Hochbaum, 1958; Estrada, 1987).
3. Stage III model variables are English language skill, knowledge of disease, and satisfaction with the health care provider.
4. Stage IV model variables are perceived health threat (severity and susceptibility), threat reduction (benefits and barriers) (Haefner et al., 1967), health locus of control (Rotter, 1954; Lau, 1982), health value orientation, and perceived treatment efficacy.
5. Stage V is outcome variable of preventive health behavior.

The causal linkages among the variables are specified with straight arrows. Correlational relationships are illustrated with curved double-arrowed lines.

Literature Review Supporting the Model

The research literature from various disciplines has shown ample evidence supporting behavioral factors as determinants of compliance and adherence (DiMatteo and DiNicola, 1982; Cummings, Becker, and Maile, 1980; Eraker, Kirscht, and Becker, 1984; Basch et al., 1983; Becker et al., 1977a; Maiman et al., 1977; Pender, 1987; Sackett and Haynes, 1976). Previous models explaining preventive behavior have included examination of the structural, situational, knowledge levels, and personal motivations toward prevention and self-efficacy (Bandura, 1977, 1982a,b).

Self-Efficacy and Treatment Efficacy

Self-efficacy is a key predictor of adherence to therapeutic or preventive regimens (Sackett and Haynes, 1976; Bandura, 1977;

1982a,b). Research by Bandura (1982a,b) substantiates that, if an individual judges him/herself to be capable of executing a given action, he/she will perform the action more proficiently. Personal efficacy is vital to performance (O'Leary, 1985), because of the cognitive-action link between underestimation of abilities and poor performance. Gilchrist and Schinke (1983) found that adolescent females with higher self-efficacy were more likely to report continued contraceptive use at the six-month evaluative follow-up. Condiotte and Lichtenstein (1981) also found a relationship between high self-efficacy and successful smoking cessation over time. Chambliss and Murray (1979) found that those who were more efficacious lost significantly more weight than either those scoring low on self-efficacy.

Self-efficacy is social in origin and may vary according to the complexity of the focal task (Kegeles and Grady, 1982; Bandura, 1977; 1982a,b). For example, taking a fiber/calcium supplement is a simple act; while introduction of fiber via dietary modification requires a more complex set of behaviors. Dietary modification encompasses new or unfamiliar food selection and purchases, meal planning and preparation, as well as negotiation with family members to cooperate. The more complex the new set of tasks, the more likely that less self-efficacious individuals will experience anxiety and resistance to adaptation (Bandura, 1982a,b).

Furthermore, self-efficacy is affected by cues from the social environment that reinforce or decrease its strength (Bandura, Adams, and Beyer, 1977; Biran and Wilson, 1981; Feltz, Landers, and Raeder, 1979). Others in the social environment reinforce the appropriateness of a given behavior, can teach or model correct behaviors and can provide feedback to affect self-efficacy (Bandura, Reese, and Adams, 1982; Gottlieb, 1981; Israel, 1982). Thus self-efficacy is postulated to be directly affected by social support.

Perceived efficacy of treatment[2] is another aspect of efficacy that is positively related to preventive health behavior (Montano, 1983). Simon (1979) found that consistent preventive behavior was reported only for those who believed the given treatment was effective in treating illness. The patient must believe that a specific disease prevention strategy will effectively prevent or cure disease before engaging in health action (Grady et al., 1983).

Social Support

Social support from familial or friendship networks can affect preventive health behavior in other ways. Social support (i.e, encouragement), can include material assistance, emotional support in the form of encouragement and feedback to correct inappropriate behavior (Gottlieb, 1981; Israel, 1982; Cassel, 1976). Research shows that positive social support provides emotional support, referrals and information (McKinlay, 1973; Granovetter, 1976), a context for learning effective coping strategies (Bloom et al., 1978; Hubbard et al., 1984), and feedback to correct inappropriate actions (Cassel, 1976). Bloom, Ross, and Burnell (1978) document the relationship of social support from the immediate kinship and friendship network(s) as predictive of adjustment to postoperative status and compliance to treatment. Heinzelmann and Bagley (1970) found that a wife's support of preventive health programs for heart disease predicted the husband's level of compliance to a special health activity program. Diamond, Weiss, and Grynbaum (1968) report that the family's support of rehabilitation is the most important factor in determining the patient's participation and compliance in spinal cord rehabilitation.

In contrast, more recent research shows that social support has costs as well as benefits. Tilden and Gaylan (1987) cite evidence from a variety of studies that document the negative effects of certain support functions on health outcomes. Many of the negative effects stem from the reciprocal obligations that ensue from receiving social support, which are perceived as a cost (e.g., guilt). Another negative effect can be the perception that one's privacy is invaded once another person in the support network has helped the individual at an emotional level. The need for adequate personal space appears to apply cross-culturally. In their study of the support functions of Mexican American families, Keefe et al. (1979) found some respondents who reported avoiding seeking emotional support in order to prevent invasion of privacy.

Health Locus of Control

Other research supports the role of health locus of control in affecting health behavior (Lau, 1982). One's perception of control as emanating from internal sources has been shown to relate positively to adherence to hypertensive treatment (Kirscht and Rosenstock, 1977), weight control programs (Chambliss and Murray, 1979), and self-selection into Breast Self-Examination (BSE) training (Grady et al., 1983).

A number of researchers propose that Mexican Americans are more likely than Anglos to believe in chance or external control (Jessor et al., 1968; Kluckhohn and Strodtbeck, 1961). The Copeland et al. (1983) study suggests that Hispanics may be less internally controlled with regard to health, as Hispanic parents in the study reported less participation in therapeutic decisions made about their childrens' cancer treatment.

Mirowsky and Ross (1984) contend that Mexican culture is related to external locus of control and hence, higher levels of depression. Developing a structural equation model (Jöreskog and Sörbom, 1986), they conclude that belief in external control was an intervening factor between Mexican culture and level of depression. However, these authors assumed that Mexican culture per se and not other factors were the cause of external control. The relationship between external control and Mexican culture could be an artifact of income, education, or other life experiences. The empirical assumptions made under LISREL were also questionable, since they did not indicate the respective t-values for the gamma and beta coefficients. Furthermore, the authors base their decisions about fixing or freeing parameters based on the standard errors of the coefficients.[3] The linkage between Mexican heritage and external locus of control may be due to impoverished status and not cultural differences (Casavantes, 1970; Garza and Ames, 1976). Copeland et al. (1983) note that lack of fluency in English is an important factor that could impede effective health care decisions. Thus, income and English language proficiency are important factors to consider as antecedents of health locus of control among Hispanics.

Health Value Orientations

Health value orientations are one's specific beliefs about the importance of health care. They are important standards on which health behavior is based and derive from one's socio-cultural milieu. Health value orientations are linked to preventive care (Murdaugh, 1982).

Castro et al. (1984) contend that Mexican American women have a dual system of health value orientations which include a reliance on traditional folk remedies and illness etiology, along with a high degree of trust in physicians, and strong acceptance of cardiovascular and stress illness concepts. These contrasting belief sets do not impede health care among Hispanics, but it is possible that decisions regarding when to use either system could possibly delay seeking of medical treatment.[4]

The Health Belief Model

The original HBM has been a central focus of compliance research. Several studies testing the HBM show that a patient's perception of disease as serious (Becker, Drachman, and Kirscht, 1972; Francis, Korsch, and Morris, 1969; Haefner and Kirscht, 1970; Kegeles, 1963; Neely and Patrick, 1968) is positively related to compliance; while other studies show no significant relationship between perception of severity and compliance (Macrae et al., 1984).

For example, Macrae et al. (1984) found that only perceived internal barriers, such as inconvenience and embarrassment, were predictive of compliance with colon cancer screening. Perceived severity and susceptibility were not significant predictors of compliance. However, validity of their measures was not identified. More recent research continues to demonstrate incomplete or contradictory findings (Calnan and Rutter, 1986); even less is known about the Hispanic population. Hence the HBM is included in the model as a predictor of preventive health behavior.

Knowledge Levels and Client/Provider Relationship

Knowledge of the disease and satisfaction with the client/provider relationship are two additional foci of the Hispanic Health Behavior in Cancer Prevention Model. Several studies show an association between knowledge of disease and compliance (Marsh and Perlman, 1972; Watkins et al., 1967), while others show no association between knowledge levels and compliance for the general population (Evans et al., 1970; Suchman, 1967).

In case studies of Mexican American pediatric heart patients and their parents, Anderson et al. (1982) found that a communication gap between Mexican American parents and the physician impeded the acceptance of diagnosis. In cases where the physician validated the parents' religious values and beliefs about treatment, he was able to reach consensus with the family and progress with appropriate treatment. These findings indicate that in the absence of sound patient/doctor communication, the physician's diagnosis will not result in patient adherence to treatment regimens.

Similarly Copeland et al. (1983) provide interesting descriptive data on Hispanics' knowledge of disease and satisfaction with the client/provider relationship. Their study assessed the attitudes of Hispanic and Anglo parents toward their childrens' cancer treatment. Significant differences between Anglo and Hispanic parents were reported regarding confidence in the physician, comfort in approaching the physician, and level of information regarding their child's disease.

Utilization Barriers

Motivation to engage in preventive behavior can be lessened by utilization barriers that impede action. These physical barriers can consist of tangible obstacles to access, lack of material resources (Bandura, 1977; 1982a), and poor environmental reinforcement. Any of these factors can constrain action.

There can be a number of specific utilization barriers that can minimize an effective cognition-action linkage for Hispanics. Utilization barriers are obstacles to access of health care, in contrast to a cognition or attitude that one might hold toward the health care system or specific treatment. Several possible barriers are the cost of preventive care, lack of transportation or childcare, and lack of Spanish-speaking staff (Marín et al., 1983). Past studies have not clearly differentiated between access barriers and internal barriers, such as those reported in Macrae et al. (1984). Preliminary work being done by Estrada (1987)[5] clearly shows cost of care and knowing where care is available to be the highest ranked barriers that prevent elderly Hispanics from getting needed care. Moreover, over 20 percent of the elderly Hispanics having some form of health insurance reported having other barriers that prevented health care. Other barriers for elderly Hispanics consisted of transportation, childcare, and institutional obstacles such as inconvenient clinic hours, long waits in the office, and excessive lag time between calling for an appointment and actually seeing the doctor. For hypertensive and diabetic Hispanics, over 80 percent of those who reported one or more barriers to care also stated that these barriers prevented them from getting needed medical care. Clearly, those Hispanics most in need of care were not receiving medical attention, regardless of cognitive or behavioral factors that might impact preventive care. Marks et al. (1987) found that access to health care and availability of services were stronger determinants of Hispanic health behavior than level of acculturation and English language proficiency. Level of acculturation and English language proficiency had a weak, but significant effect on health behavior. These data clearly suggest that access barriers are distinct from individual level barriers, such as fear and embarrassment, or inconvenience of treatment. The behavioral model presented here separates the two types of barriers and places physical barriers to utilization as antecedent to internal barriers. In this way, the distinct impact of types of barriers can be assessed in empirical tests of the model.

Demographic Background as a Predictor of Preventive Health Behavior

Finally, based on this previous work, background social characteristics are predicted to affect preventive health behavior. Rosenstock's (1974) research documents that there is a positive relationship between delay in seeking diagnosis and socioeconomic status. Persons who delay tend to be older, less affluent members of ethnic minority groups, and/or male. Socioeconomic status, marital status, and acculturation level are predicted to have differential effects on preventive health behavior through intervening variables such as English language proficiency, health status, and social support. For example, Richardson et al. (1987) in their study of 600 elderly Mexican American women found that refusal to participate in a simulated breast self-examination was related to age and level of acculturation. Among those who participated, proficiency in locating lumps in the breast model was positively related to younger age and higher level of acculturation, which in turn were related to greater English language proficiency.

POLICY IMPLICATIONS

The National Cancer Institute supports the goal of a 50-percent reduction in cancer incidence by the year 2000. A specific program objective is to focus on the relationship between knowledge, attitudes and beliefs, and health care behavior among Hispanics (Proceedings Summary of the Hispanic Cancer Control Program Workshop, 1986). Understanding cultural differences in how individuals process health information and subsequently act upon it is critical to changing unhealthy habits or introducing long-term health promoting behaviors. Understanding of the social, cultural, and behavioral factors that facilitate or impede Hispanics' health behavior will enable effective structuring of educational programs in the Hispanic community. The identification and ranking of specific barriers to health care and their relationship to preventive health behavior will enable policy makers and care providers to design appropriate interventions in the Hispanic community. Informed policy making based on theory and its application can facilitate early diagnosis, successful treatment, and lower incidence rates for particular diseases. However, until researchers and policy makers understand how individuals are motivated to seek health care, gains in treatment technology will remain unproductive in reducing morbidity and mortality for certain populations.

REFERENCE NOTES

1. Hispanic refers to all Spanish-origin persons residing in the United States. Mexican American refers to Mexican-origin persons exclusively. Terms are used as they appear in cited works.

2. Efficacy of treatment refers to the belief that a given treatment or course of action will effectively prevent disease or cure it (Bandura, 1977;1982a).

3. Large standard errors relative to estimated coefficients may be due to measurement error as opposed to model estimation error, hence, it is advisable to

base decisions about fixing or freeing parameters on the t-values, modification indices, and the theoretical model being tested.

4. Unpublished ethnographic work being done by Mr. Robert Dalgarn, Northern Arizona University among Tucson Hispanic males indicates that these men employ a decision-making system that proceeds from ignoring symptoms to use of home remedies when symptoms persist, to seeking help from female significant others at the point when they perceive a given illness to be uncontrollable. Only when these avenues fail, do they seek medical attention. The definition of an illness as controllable versus uncontrollable seems to be the fulcrum point between two incongruent health belief systems. Whether females use the same system is debatable.

5. Dr. Estrada, of the Rural Health Office, University of Arizona is currently researching barriers to utilization of health care among elderly Hispanics (over 50). His data stem from the Hispanic Health and Nutrition Examination Survey conducted in the Southwest, New York City, and Miami during 1982-84. His analysis focuses on the Mexican American database, although data is now available for Puerto Ricans and Cubans.

REFERENCES

Anderson, B.G., Toledo, J.R., Hazam, N. (1982). An approach to the resolution of Mexican American resistance to diagnostic and remedial pediatric heart care. In *Clinical Applied Anthropology*, edited by J. Christman and T.W. Maretzki (pp. 325-350). D. Reidel Publishing Company.

Atwood, J.R. (1986). Conceptualization: Concept development, the progress to quantification. *Proceedings of the 3rd Annual Nursing Science Colloquium.* 37-66, Boston, Boston University School of Nursing.

Bandura A. (1977). Self-efficacy: Toward a unifying theory of behavioral change. *Psychological Review, 84*, 191-215.

Bandura, A. (1982a). The self and mechanisms of agency. In *Psychological perspectives on the self*, edited by Jerry Suls. Lawrence Erlbaum Associates.

Bandura, A. (1982b). Self-efficacy mechanism in human agency. *American Psychologist, 37*(2), 122-147.

Bandura, A., Adams, N.E., & Beyer, J. (1977). Cognitive processes mediating behavioral change. *Journal of Personality and Social Psychology, 35*, 125-139.

Bandura, A., Reese, L., & Adams, N.E. (1982). Microanalysis of action and fear arousal as a function of differential levels of perceived self-efficacy. *Journal of Personality and Social Psychology, 43*(1), 5-21.

Basch, C.E., Gold, R.F., McDermott, R.J., & Richardson, C.E. (1983). Confounding variables in the measurement of cancer patient compliance. *Cancer Nursing, 6*, 4, 285-293.

Becker, M.H., Drachman, R.H., & Kirscht, J.P. (1972). Motivations as predictors of health behavior. *Health Services Rep., 87*, 852-61.

Becker, M.H., Maiman, L.A., Kirscht, J.P., Haefner, D.P., & Drachman, R.H.

(1977a). The health belief model and prediction of dietary compliance: A field experiment. *Journal of Health and Social Behavior*, 8, 348-366.

Belloc, N.B., & Breslow, L. (1972). Relationship of physical health status and health practices. *Preventive Medicine, 1*, 409-421.

Biran M., & Wilson, G.T. (1981). Cognitive versus behavioral methods in the treatment of phobic disorders: A self-efficacy analysis. *Journal of Consulting and Clinical Psychology*, 886-889.

Bloom, J.R., Ross, R.D., & Burnell, G.M. (1978). Effect of social support on patient adjustment following surgery. *Patient Counseling and Health Education*, 1:50-59.

Calnan, M.W., & Moss, S. (Eds.) (1984, July). The health belief model and compliance with education given at a class in breast self-examination. *Journal of Health and Social Behavior, 25*, 198-210.

Calnan, M. & Rutter, D.R. (1986). Do health beliefs predict health behavior? An analysis of breast self-examination. *Social Science in Medicine, 22*, 6, 673-718.

Casavantes, E. (Winter 1970). Pride and prejudice: A Mexican American dilemma. *Civil Rights Digest, 3*, 22-27.

Cassel, J. (1976). The contribution of the social environment to host resistance. *American Journal of Epidemiology*, 104:107-123.

Castro, F.G., Furth, P., & Karlon, H. (1984). The health beliefs of Mexican, Mexican Americans, and Anglo American women. *Hispanic Journal of Behavioral Sciences, 6*, 365-383.

Chambliss, C.A., & Murray, E.J. (1979). Efficacy attribution, locus of control and weight loss. *Cognitive Therapy and Research, 3*(4), 349-353.

Condiotte, M.M., & Lichtenstein, E. (1981). Self-efficacy and relapse in smoking cessation programs. *Journal of Consulting Psychology, 49*, 648-658.

Copeland, D.R., Silberberg, Y., & Pfefferbaum, B. (Spring 1983). Attitudes and practices of families of children in treatment for cancer: A cross-cultural study. *American Journal of Pediatric Hematology and Oncology, 5*(1), 65-71.

Cummings, K.M., Becker, M.H., & Maile, M.C. (1980). Bringing the models together: An empirical approach to combining variables used to explain health actions. *Journal of Behavioral Medicine, 3*(2), 123-145.

Daly, M.B., Clark, G.M., & McGuire, W.L. (1985, April). Breast cancer prognosis in a mixed Caucasian-Hispanic population: 1971-1982 study data. *Journal of the National Cancer Institute, 74*(4), 753-757.

Diamond, M.D., Weiss, A.J., & Grynbaum, B. (1968). The unmotivated patient. *Archives of Physical Medicine and Rehabilitation, 49*, 281-284.

DiMatteo, M.R., & DiNicola, D.D. (1982). *Achieving patient compliance: The psychology of the medical practitioners' role*. New York: Pergamon Press.

Eraker, S.A., Kirscht, J.P., & Becker, M.H. (1984). Understanding and improving patient compliance. *Annals of Internal Medicine, 100*, 258-268.

Estrada, T. (1987, May). Barriers to utilization among Mexican Americans: Evidence from HHANES. Unpublished paper presented at the Arizona/Chicano Conference.

Evans, R.I., Rozelle, R.M., Lasater, T.M., Dembroski, T.M., and Allen, B.P. (1970). Fear arousal, persuasion, and actual versus implied behavioral change. *J. Personality and Soc. Psychol., 16*, 220-227.

Feltz, D.L., Landers, D.M., & Raeder, V. (1979). Enhancing self-efficacy in high-avoidance motor tasks: A comparison of modeling techniques. *Journal of Sport Psychology, 1*, 112-122.

Francis, V., Korsch, B.M., & Morris, M.J. (1969). Gaps in doctor-patient communication. *New England Journal of Medicine, 280*, 535-40.

Garza, R.T., & Ames, R.E. (1976). A comparison of Chicanos and Anglos on locus of control. In C.A. Hernandez, M.J. Haug, and N.N. Wagner (Eds.) *Chicanos: Social and psychological perspectives.* (2nd Ed.) C.V. Mosby.

Gilchrist, L.D., & Schinke, S.P. (1983). Coping with contraception: Cognitive and behavioral methods with adolescents. *Cognitive Therapy and Research, 7*(5), 379-388.

Gottlieb, B.H. (1981). Social networks and social support in community mental health. In *Social networks and social support,* edited by B.H. Gottlieb. Beverly Hills: Sage Publications.

Grady, K.E., Kegeles, S.S., Lund, A.K., Wolk, C.H., & Farber, N.J. (Summer 1983). Who volunteers for a breast self-examination? Evaluating the bases for self-selection. *Health Education Quarterly, 10*(2), 79-94.

Granovetter, M.S. (1976). The strength of weak ties. *American Journal of Sociology, 78*: 1360-1380.

Haefner, D.P., & Kirscht, J.P. (1970). Motivational and behavioral effects of modifying health beliefs. *Public Health Reports, 85*, 478-84.

Haefner, D.P., Kegeles, S.S., Kirscht, J., & Rosenstock, I.M. (1967, May). Preventive actions in dental disease, tuberculosis, and cancer. *Public Health Reports, 82*(5), 451-459.

Heinzelmann, F. & Bagley, R. W. (1970). Response to physical activity programs and their effects on health behavior. *Public Health Reports, 85*(10), 905-911.

Hershey, J.C., Morton, B.G., Davis, J.B., & Reichgott, M.J. (1980). Patient compliance with antihypertensive medication. *American Journal of Public Health, 70*, 10, 1081-1089.

Hindi-Alexander, M.C. & Throm, J. (1987). Compliance or non-compliance: That is the question! *American Journal of Health Promotion. 1*(4):5-11.

Hochbaum, G.M. (1958). Public participation in Medical screening programs: A Social psychological study. Public Health Service, Public Health Service Publication No. 572, Washington, United States Government Printing Office.

Hubbard, P., Muhlenkamp, A.F., & Brown, N. (1984, October). The relationship between social support and self-care practices. *Nursing Research, 33*(5), 266-270.

Israel, B.A. (1982). Social networks and health status: Linking theory, research and practice. *Patient Counseling and Health Education, 4*, 65-79.

Janz, N.K., & Becker, M. (1984). The health belief model: A decade later. *Health Education Quarterly, 11*, 1-47.

Jessor, R., Graves, D.T., Hanson, R.C., & Jessor, S.L. (1968). *Society personality and deviant behavior.* New York: Holt, Rinehart, & Winston.

Jöreskog, K., & Sörbom, D. (1986). LISREL VI Scientific Software, Inc.

Kasl, S.V., & Cobb, S. (1986, February). Health behavior, illness behavior and sick role behavior. *Archives of Environmental Health I, 12,* 246-266 and II (1966, April). *12,* 534-541.

Keefe, S., Padilla, A., & Carlos, M. (1979). The Mexican American family as an emotional support system. *Human Organization, 38,* 3, Summer, 144-152.

Kegeles, S.S. (1963). Some motives for seeking preventive dental care. *Journal of the American Dental Association, 67,* 90-98.

Kegeles, S.S., & Grady, K.E. (1982). Behavioral dimensions. In D. Schottenfeld & J. Fraumini, J. (Eds.). *Cancer epidemiology and prevention,* (pp. 1049-1063). Philadelphia: W.B. Saunders Company.

Kirscht, J.P. & Rosenstock, I.M. (1977). Patient adherence to antihypertensive medical regimens. *Journal of Community Health, 3:*115-124.

Kluckhohn, F.R., & Strodtbeck, F.L. (1961). *Variations in Value Orientation.* Westport, CT: Greenwood Press.

Lau, R.R. (1982). Origins of health locus of control beliefs. *Journal of Personality and Social Psychology, 42(2):*322-334.

Mack, T.M., Walker, A., Mack, W., & Bernstein, L. (1985). Cancer in Hispanics in Los Angeles County. National Cancer Institute Monograph 69, 99-104.

Macrae, F.A., Hill, D.J., St. John, K.J.B., Ambikapathy, A., Garner, J.R., & the Ballarat General Practitioner Research Group. (1984). Predicting colon cancer screening behavior from health beliefs. *Preventive Medicine, 13,* 115-126.

Maiman, L.A., Becker, M.H., Kirscht, J.P., Haefner, D.P., & Drachman, R.H. (1977). Scales for measuring health belief model dimensions: A test of predictive value, internal consistency, and relationships among beliefs. *Health Education Monographs, 5(3),* 215-230.

Marin, B.V.O., Marín, G., Padilla, A., & de la Rocha, C. (1983). Utilization of traditional and non-traditional sources of health care among Hispanics. *Hispanic Journal Behavioral Sciences, 5,* 1, 65-80.

Marks, G., Solis, J., Richardson, J.L., Collins, L.M., Birba, L., & Hisserich, J.C. (1987). Health behavior of elderly Hispanic women: Does cultural assimilation make a difference? *American Journal of Public Health, 77(10),* 1315-1319.

Marsh, W.W., & Perlman, L.V. (1972). Understanding congestive heart failure and self-administration of digoxin. *Geriatrics, 27,* 65-70.

McKinlay, J.B. (1972). Some approaches and problems in the study of the use of services: An overview. *Journal of Health and Social Behavior, 13,* 115-152.

McKinlay, J.B. (1973). Social networks, law consultation, and help-seeking behavior. *Social Forces, 51,* 275-295.

Mirowsky, J., & Ross, C.E. (1984, March). Mexican culture and its emotional contradictions. *Journal of Health and Social Behavior, 25,* 2-13.

Montano, D.E. (1983). Compliance with health care recommendations: A reassessment of the health belief model. *Dissertation Abstracts International, 44(4-B),* 1281-1282.

Murdaugh, C.L. (1982). Instrument development in preventive behaviors for CAD. *Dissertation Abstracts International, 43*(3), 680b.

Neely, E., & Patrick, M.L. (1968). Problems of aged persons taking medications at home. *Nursing Research, 17*, 52-55.

O'Leary, A. (1985). Self-efficacy and health. *Behavioral Research and Therapy, 23*(4), 437-451.

Pender, N.J. (1987). *Health promotion in nursing practice.* Connecticut: Appleton-Century-Croft.

Proceedings Summary of the Hispanic Cancer Control Program Workshop, National Cancer Institute, Division of Cancer Prevention and Control (April 17-18,1986).

Richardson, J.L., Marks, G., Solis, J.M., Collins, L.M., Birba, L., & Hisserich, J.C. (1987). Frequency and adequacy of breast cancer screening among elderly Hispanic women. *Preventive Medicine, 16*, 761-774.

Rosenstock, I.M. (1974). Historical origins of health belief model. *Health Education Monographs, 2*(4), 328-335.

Rotter, J.B. (1954). *Social learning and clinical psychology.* New York: Prentice-Hall.

Sackett, D.L. & Haynes, R.B. (1976). *Compliance with therapeutic regimens.* Baltimore: The Johns Hopkins University Press.

Samet, J.M., Rey, C.R., Hunt, W.C., & Goodwin, J.S. (1987, September). Survival of American Indian and Hispanic cancer patients in New Mexico and Arizona, 1969-82. *Journal of the National Cancer Institute, 79*(3), 457-463.

Savitz, D. (1986, October). Changes in Spanish surname cancer rates relative other whites, Denver area, 1969-1971 to 1979-81. *American Journal of Public Health, 76*(10), 1210-1215.

Simon, K.M., (1979). Self-evaluative reactions: The role of personal validation of the activity. *Cognitive Therapy and Research, 3* (1A), 111-116.

Suchman, E.A. (1967) Preventive health behavior: A model for research in community health campaigns. *J. Health Soc. Behav., 8*, 197-209.

Tilden, V.P. & Gaylan, R.D. (1987). Cost and conflict: The darker side of social support. *Western Journal of Nursing Research, 9*, 1:9-18.

Watkins, J.D., Williams, T.F., Martin, D.A., Hogan, M.D., & Anderson, E. (1967). A study of diabetic patients at home. *American Journal of Public Health, 57*, 452-59.

Watts, R.J. (1982). Sexual functioning, health beliefs, and compliance with high blood pressure medications. *Nursing Research, 31*, 5, 178-183.

Chapter 18

AIDS and FDA Drug-Approval Policy:
An Evolving Controversy

Stephen J. Gould

SUMMARY. AIDS treatment policy has become controversial in recent years as the Gay AIDS Movement has challenged FDA drug-testing and approval policies. Based on the Social Movements Model (Frierson, 1985) this movement has reached the stage of establishing a compelling trend of public pressure and is moving toward the stage of the enactment of policy change. Gays have demanded a number of changes in clinical trials and other FDA rules such as the creation of community-based trials, changes in the clinical protocols, and the increased availability of experimental drugs. The FDA has made a number of changes in response, but many of the most controversial demands of the Gay community and their medical allies remain open to debate. The implications and conclusions for the possible outcomes of this controversy are considered.

INTRODUCTION

Public health policy concerning AIDS treatment has become controversial in recent years along with many other aspects of the disease. The controversy has pitted Gay groups and their advocates against the Food and Drug Administration (FDA) in a debate over drug-testing procedures, and also over the availability of new experimental (investigational) AIDS drugs (Booth, 1988; Smith and Long, 1988). This chapter considers the debate in terms of the

This chapter was originally published in *Journal of Health & Social Policy*, Vol. 2(2) 1990.

following: (1) examination of the Gay AIDS Movement as a social movement, (2) the issues this movement has raised and how the FDA has been responding, and (3) some conclusions concerning the future directions and implications of this debate.

THE GAY AIDS MOVEMENT

In confronting AIDS both in terms of prevention and treatment, the Gay community has acted in concert. Gays have drawn on their already established network of Gay groups (e.g., the National Gay and Lesbian Task Force) as well as forming specific AIDS-related groups (e.g., People with AIDS [PWA]; AIDS Coalition to Unleash Power [ACTUP]). These groups have come to directly challenge FDA policy with which they disagree and to represent Gay AIDS victims in an advocacy role. When viewed as a whole, these groups along with allied health care advocates and practitioners may be said to comprise a social movement or collectivity which acts to promote some form of social change (Turner and Killian, 1957).

In order to position the present standing of the Gay AIDS Movement, we can use the Social Movements Model which includes six stages or phases which reflect how a social problem progressively evolves into a public policy concern (Frierson, 1985). These phases include: (1) existence of the problem, (2) recognition of the problem with a few advocates for some remediation, (3) the establishment of a trend of public pressure, (4) the enactment of important legal or procedural changes, (5) enforcement of these changes, and (6) the acceptance and internalization of these changes by other institutions and individuals in society. It would appear that the Gay AIDS Movement has clearly established itself in phase 3; has established a recognizable and strong public presence in advocating greater say for itself in the scientific and medical policies of the FDA with respect to drug policy. The movement is more properly described, perhaps, as actually being in transition from phase 3 into phase 4. It has already achieved some major changes in FDA rules, such as being allowed to import experimental drugs from foreign countries through the mail (Boffey, 1988) and also the enactment by California of its own more liberalized drug-testing program. However, the movement is still more in phase 3 than 4 because most of the major Gay demands are still unmet and many remain controversial.

DRUG TESTING AND AVAILABILITY ISSUES

General Background Influencing Gay Demands

While the Gay AIDS Movement has been particularly compelling and innovative, its behavior is reflective of some larger social trends in health care. First, the public has come to take on a larger role in scientific decisions concerning health matters (Burger, 1988). Second, the patient has come to be viewed as a "consumer" of health care, a role reflective of the individual being more active than passive in the health care process. Third, many people have been active in challenging expert authority in health care as well as in other arenas of life (Ferguson, 1980; Gould, 1988). While these trends are by no means totally pervasive, and since only some segments of the population may be said to be strongly affected by them, they nonetheless do set the context for the Gay AIDS Movement which has perhaps carried these trends to their zenith. Gays have been particularly forceful in making their demands not only because of their network of interest groups mentioned above, but also because of their high levels of education, income, and professional managerial status (Kneale, 1989). Status is important because higher status individuals are more likely to receive and assimilate health information than lower status individuals and also are more likely to be complainers with respect to product or service problems (Morgansky and Buckley, 1987; Waitzkin, 1985).

The Specific Demands of the Gay AIDS Movement

We will focus here on the demands Gays have made with respect to drug-testing procedures and experimental drug availability. To be sure, they are also making a demand for more research money in general, but this is a rather universal demand which most advocates for research into any disease are likely to make. What differentiates and distinguishes the Gay AIDS Movement are its other demands.

The Gay community has felt that the development of new AIDS drugs has lagged and that FDA approval procedures have been largely to blame. It has been claimed that too few new drugs have been tested, that there is no coordinated national program of testing, that information regarding the results of clinical trials is slow in being disseminated, and that FDA rules and procedures are not clear to health care practitioners and pharmaceutical companies (Smith and Long, 1988). Gays also cite the large numbers of experimental drugs which are available on the "underground" market as an impetus for matters to be speeded up. They have suggested that there be increased clinical trial access and also changes in the clinical trial procedures, themselves, which would facilitate the quality of their medical care (Smith and Long, 1988).

With respect to increasing clinical trials, Gays have suggested running their own community-based trials with interested physicians in their own communities. In response to such demands, the FDA has moved to encourage more community-based trials (Altman, 1988). Finally, Gays have also demanded greater access to whatever experimental drugs are available, including those from abroad (Boffey, 1988). The FDA has responded by increasing their access and will look to monitor these in efficiency through community-based programs as well (Altman, 1988; Clark and Hager, 1988).

More controversial and complex are the demands concerned with changes in the testing procedures, themselves. Gay advocates, such as Mathilde Krim, have long argued that alternative ways to test drugs might be used to eliminate use of inactive placebos in trials (Chase, 1986; Smith and Long, 1988). Providing dying patients with placebos is unethical because they should be getting something which at least has a chance of helping them. The FDA has responded so far by speeding up procedures in order to make investigational drugs available more quickly to patients. For example, it has acted so that broad phase 3 clinical studies may be bypassed in the case of life-threatening or debilitating diseases (Marwick, 1988; Young et al., 1988).

However many are still in doubt about what to expect from the FDA. Recently, for example, controversy has risen over the drug gangciclovir which has been licensed for "compassionate use" to prevent blindness from cytomegalovirus in AIDS patients (Kolata,

1988). The drug, which has already been approved in England, France, Belgium, and Holland, has been found by many physicians in the U.S. to be successful in treating cytomegalovirus. Yet, the FDA decided to restrict the use of the drug until further controlled testing is done. They did make exemptions for those already using the drug, but many feel that this additional testing is completely unnecessary. More recently, the FDA, in response to pressure from AIDS-patient advocates, has moved in the direction of reversing itself and broadening the use of gangciclovir (Chase, 1989).

In addition to doubts about how the FDA will administer its current policies, others have expressed concerns about the nature of the policy in more fundamental terms. A former head of the FDA, Dr. Jere Goyan (1988) feels that much more than tinkering with the system is needed. He has called for the development of new testing protocols in which patients would all get some sort of potentially helpful substance rather than a placebo in their trials. They would then be randomly assigned to treatment protocols which excluded placebos. There would be no guarantee as to what substance they would be receiving but they would know that they would be getting an investigational drug from a known list of those drugs. While Goyan admits there might be less security in the findings, there would be greater ease in doing the studies because of better patient cooperation which has been lacking in recent clinical trials for AIDS drugs. Such types of trials, he feels, would increase the patient's sense of self-determination while retaining scientific control as well.

CONCLUSIONS

The Gay AIDS Social Movement has precipitated major controversy over FDA testing procedures which may have effects which spill over into the domains of other diseases. For instance, other groups may demand greater access to investigational drugs as well. To the degree that this social movement succeeds in its goals and perhaps to the degree that AIDS comes to threaten our whole society, we may come to recognize ourselves as being in the midst of a paradigm shift (Kuhn, 1970) with respect to drug-testing policy and investigational drug availability. While it is very difficult to predict how these issues will play themselves out, there are several things which we should look for in making public health decisions in this area:

- Gays will continue to press for changes in government policy with respect to drug testing and approval procedures. They are likely to be joined in these demands by others over time should AIDS spread to other well-educated segments of the population, just as they have already been joined by many health care practitioners.
- As the population gets better educated and older, more people will take an increasing interest in their health and are more likely to be a part of public pressure groups for particular diseases or even preventive health causes, especially if the Gay AIDS Movement continues to set a precedent.
- While some groups will seek a greater voice and participation, other segments of the population, such as the poor, less educated, and children may require different sorts of policies; a blanket mass-policy with respect to investigational drugs does not seem as desirable as one which assesses different diseases and different demographic groups differently. This requires the use of what is called "market segmentation," which is the identification of markets or groups of patients with similar needs and demographic, lifestyle, and disease characteristics (Schiffman and Kanuk, 1987). The identification of such segments can be an important step in designing drug-approval interventions which are targeted for specific groups and therefore are more likely to be effective in achieving promotion of overall public health. The FDA is already doing this in part by singling out AIDS for high priority and by characterizing it as different from other diseases.
- Policy makers will need to find a new equilibrium in the balance between preventing unsafe drugs from penetrating the clinical marketplace (a Type I error in statistical terms), on the one hand, and missing opportunities to provide truly efficacious drugs for needy patients (a Type II error), on the other (Neter, Wasserman, and Whitmore, 1978). For many AIDS victims, the present risks of Type II errors are too great.

Finding equilibrium in this regard will not be easy, but perhaps by looking at different diseases and populations individually as suggested in the previous point, policy makers may come to vary the risks they allow across different groups (e.g., pregnant women versus terminal AIDS patients). Striking a balance between compassion and knowledge has never been an easy dilemma to face and has been made perhaps even more difficult in the face of the demands of the AIDS epidemic.

- Concerned citizens should be included on a much more formal basis in scientific policy making which involves their own interests than they have been in the past. Such involvement may take the form of advisory panels, consumer surveys, and community-based participation in trials.

The AIDS crisis is causing us to take a new look at our scientific procedures regarding drug safety and efficacy. Ultimately, what we do in this regard will have implications for all patients, no matter what disease they have.

REFERENCES

Altman, L.K. (1988). F.D.A. approves first drug for an AIDS-related cancer. *The New York Times*, November 22, C3.

Boffey, P.M. (1988). Importing AIDS drugs: Analysis of F.D.A. policy. *The New York Times*, July 26, C1, C6.

Booth, W. (1988). AIDS policy in the making. *Science*, March 4, 1987.

Burger, Jr. E.J. (1988). Scientific information in judicial and administrative systems. *Social Science and Medicine*, 27, 1031-1041.

Chase, M. (1986). AIDS research stirs bitter fight over use of experimental drugs. *Wall Street Journal*, June 18, 29.

Chase, M. (1989). Drug for blindness linked to AIDS is kept off market due to miscues. *Wall Street Journal*, February 10, B2.

Clark, M. & Hager, M. (1988). The drug-approval dilemma: Does FDA mean foot-dragging administration? *Newsweek*, November 14, 63.

Ferguson, T. (1980). Medical self-care: Self-responsibility for health. In *Health for the Whole Person*, edited by A.C. Hastings, J.F. Fadiman, & J.S. Gordon, Boulder, CO: Westview.

Frierson J.G. (1985). Public policy forecasting: A new approach. *Advanced Management Journal*, 50, 18-23.

Gould, S.J. (1988). Consumer attitudes toward health and health care: A differential perspective. *Journal of Consumer Affairs*, 22, 96-118.

Goyan, J.E. (1988). Drug regulation: Quo vadis. *Journal of the American Medical Association*, 260, 3052-3053.

Kneale, D. (1989). Advertising: Gay consumer spending. *Wall Street Journal*, February 10, B3.

Kolata, G. (1988). Despite promise in AIDS Cases, drug faces testing hurdle. *The New York Times*, December 13, C3.

Kuhn, T.S. (1970). *The Structure of Scientific Revolutions*. Chicago: University of Chicago Press.

Marwick, C. (1988). FDA seeks swifter approval of drugs for some life-threatening or debilitating diseases. *Journal of the American Medical Association*, 260, 2976.

Morgansky M.A. & Buckley, H.M. (1987). Complaint behavior: Analysis by demographics, lifestyle, and consumer values. In Advances in Consumer Research, edited by Melanie Wallendorf and Paul Anderson. Vol. 14. Provo, UT: Association for Consumer Research.

Neter, J., Wasserman W., & Whitmore, G.A. (1978). *Applied Statistics*. Boston: Allyn and Bacon.

Schiffman, L.G., & Kanuk L.L. (1987). *Consumer Behavior*, Third Edition. Englewood Cliffs, NJ: Prentice-Hall.

Smith, K. & Long, I. (1988). New York State AIDS Treatment Evaluation Units Progress Report. New York: ACTUP (AIDS Coalition to Unleash Power).

Turner, R.H. & Killian, L.M. (1957). *Collective Behavior*, Englewood Cliffs, NJ: Prentice-Hall.

Waitzkin, H. (1985). Information giving in medical care. *Journal of Health and Social Behavior*, 26,81-101.

Young, F.E., Norris, J.A., Levitt, J.A., & Nightengale, S.L. (1988). The FDA's new procedures for the use of investigational drugs in treatment. *Journal of the American Medical Association*, 259, 2267-2270.

Index